To the Memory of

SIR HUGH CAIRNS

pioneer of crash helmets for motor-cyclists;

and

to my other teachers.

The Practical Management of Head Injuries

JOHN M. POTTER

M.A. (Cantab.), D.M. (Oxon.), F.R.C.S.

Director of Postgraduate Medical Education and Training, University of Oxford; University Lecturer in Neurosurgery and Fellow of Wadham College; Honorary Consultant Neurosurgeon, United Oxford Hospitals and Oxford Regional Hospital Board; formerly Consultant Neurosurgeon to the Manchester Royal Infirmary and Manchester Regional Hospital Board; and Clinical Lecturer in Neurosurgery, University of Manchester.

Third Edition

LLOYD-LUKE (MEDICAL BOOKS) LTD
49 NEWMAN STREET
LONDON
1974

First Edition . . . 1961
Reprinted 1963
Second Edition . . 1964
Reprinted 1968
Third Edition . . . 1974

PRINTED AND BOUND IN ENGLAND BY
HAZELL WATSON AND VINEY LTD
AYLESBURY, BUCKS

ISBN 0 85324 108 2

. . . there are many disorders strictly within the surgeon's province, the management of which will require more real skill, and judgment, than are necessary for the mere performance of any operation whatever;

PERCIVALL POTT, 1760

FOREWORD

THOUGH many lives are lost through head injuries a considerable proportion of them could have been saved by prompt and judicious treatment. To most recently qualified practitioners examination of the nervous system is a lengthy process which seems to be reliable only when it is done by a specialist, yet the proper examination of a patient after a head injury demands a knowledge of what to look for rather than great neurological expertise. Neurosurgery has come to be regarded as a specialty requiring such judgement and training that it can be successfully practised only by a select few; yet the management of head injuries, especially in the acute phase, is well within the competence of the general surgeon. It is to place head injuries in their proper perspective, to dispel the superstitious fear that they engender, and to give the necessary guidance to those who are called upon to deal with them that this book has been written. It makes an honest attempt to tackle an urgent problem in a practical way, and anyone who reads it carefully must agree that its objective has been achieved.

It must not be supposed from these introductory remarks that the author underestimates the serious nature of head injuries—on the contrary, the gravity and the frequency of these accidents are fully recognized. Furthermore, the reasons for segregating the victims of cerebral injury in special units, and the important part to be played by surgeons expert in neurological problems are convincingly presented. Nevertheless, it is its straightforward, methodical approach to the subject, and the obvious intention to give advice in a simple, clear, and concise form that must make the most direct appeal to the inexpert.

To say that the book has the virtue of being based on experience is but half the truth; it is founded also upon sound physiology and careful clinical methods. The author's quality as a teacher is shown by his ability to distinguish clearly between the more and the less important aspects of the subject; and his discrimination in the use of emphasis gives the book a vitality characteristic of the spoken rather than of the written word. Those who know Mr. Potter well can listen to him saying what they read. What he has written deserves to be read by all who have to treat accidents; and being short it is as easy as it is profitable to read it over and over again. As for myself I have appreciated the opportunity of reading the book and the invitation to write this foreword.

J. PATERSON ROSS

PREFACE TO THE THIRD EDITION

THIS is only one of many possible systems for dealing with injuries of the head. It is intended to be a practical guide and is not designed to help those who wish merely to pass surgical examinations. Those who work under satisfactory conditions may not appreciate the emphasis attached to certain sections, because I have tried to have always in mind those who practise in the smaller hospitals to which so many head injuries are at present taken, but where the arrangements are often far from suitable for this type of case.

As an individual approach to the subject, this book can, I am well aware, be criticized on many scores: the arrangement and emphasis, for example, are such that it does not follow a conventional pattern. Moreover, it has been necessary, in so small a space, to compress a great deal of factual information, so that some important points may not stand out as perhaps they should. But the object of a book is that it should be read, and I have done my best to avoid the dullness that is so apt to result from condensation, hoping that I have managed to convey to the reader the attitude of mind that is so necessary for head-injury work—a combination of alertness, anticipation, well-directed energy and a sense of urgency.

In the Appendix entitled, "Lost Bouquets", Brian Elliott describes what it means to lose one's sense of smell. I have included this unusual item because I do not think that it is sufficiently appreciated what a tragic disability anosmia can be, and I hope that readers will be grateful with me to Mr. Elliott and the B.B.C. for their permission to reproduce what was originally a radio broadcast. And, to illustrate the easily performed test for positional vertigo (an organic symptom often mistaken for a neurotic one), Dr. C. S. Hallpike's charming and already much published diagram (Fig. 8) has been reproduced by permission of the editor of the *Postgraduate Medical Journal.*

I have again been grateful to many reviewers. In attempting both to meet their kindly criticisms of the previous edition and to bring this book up to date, I have been restrained only by my persisting belief that it should be possible to write all that is really needed in less than one hundred pages. The basic principles of management have not changed, and new knowledge has yet to become firmly enough established to warrant their modification. For example, the continuous monitoring of changes in intracranial pressure, which has been carried out in certain specialized units, appears so far to have added more to our knowledge of these changes than to the understanding of their significance in relation to treatment.

It remains more of a problem, however, to provide an organization capable of delivering the fruits of our knowledge.

'Intensive Care'

'Intensive care' has always been an essential part of neurosurgical practice, inseparable from the development of the specialty and from the satisfactory treatment of patients with head and other injuries. That this synonym for such proper care should have become something of a cliché is a result of the difficulty of providing sufficient nurses to give this care to all patients requiring modern methods of treatment of increasing complexity. But if nursing policy requires that all intensive care should be concentrated on one area, it must still be recognized that there is a need there for specialist nursing as much as for medical expertise in different fields. The care of patients with head injuries is a case in point: this is not appropriately given by those who, however expert in, say, the management of respiratory insufficiency, do not know enough about head injuries.

Three main systems of providing for the intensive care of the injured may be recognized. In the first, the patients are in the charge of a doctor trained essentially in one particular aspect of injury, probably an orthopaedic surgeon or an anaesthetist. In the second system, a form of committee-care is liable to prevail, in which each specialty deals with its own problem. This is insufficiently responsible to the whole patient unless personal relationships and communications between specialties are of a high order. But if efficiently combined with the first system or, better, with that to be described next, this method may work well. But, as specialties multiply and become more independent and intellectually isolated from one another, it becomes increasingly difficult to achieve satisfactory co-ordination. The third system, therefore, is to have in administrative charge a doctor with *sufficient* general knowledge of *all* aspects of injury to act as a co-ordinator among those whose special knowledge is available for the different injuries. It is my hope that, in this way, 'general surgery', which now survives in little more than its still prestigious name, may yet be reborn in relation to the surgery of trauma.

To my masters and former colleagues my gratitude is no less now than when it was recorded in the two earlier editions: Sir James Paterson Ross, John O'Connell, Joe Pennybacker, Richard Johnson, Walpole Lewin, J. C. Scott, Harold Bolton, Edward Anderson, Anthony Anscombe, Bryan Jennett, J. A. H. Henderson, Robert Ollerenshaw and Sister Ruth Martin, M.B.E.

Now, further acknowledgements of loyalty and support are due. To Sister Ann Thompson and to a succession of registrars I am much in debt. Richard Gye, who has taken over administrative charge of the department of neurosurgery at Oxford, Edward Hitchcock, Denis Keown, David Budd, Tom Fisher, Michael Briggs, Nigel Tubbs, Donald Shaw and Dave Mohan have all contributed to the changes made in this edition. Lastly, I should record the patience shown by my publisher, Mr. Douglas Luke, while I allowed this book to go out of print during its revision.

J. M. P.

Oxford,
April, 1974

CONTENTS

Chapter 1

INTRODUCTION

It is unfortunate that man has difficulty in learning much from wars. Important lessons about head injuries were taught during the last war by those such as Cairns, Symonds and Ritchie Russell who were in the Armed Services, and by Jefferson, Dott and Rowbotham in the Emergency Medical Service at home. These medical and surgical neurologists showed what could be achieved by an organized head injury service. Yet now there is no sufficiently widespread policy for the efficient treatment of these cases and some feel that there has been retrogression.

There has been no lack of instruction. The urgency of the treatment of extradural haemorrhage, for example, and the means of identifying and arresting this thief in the night, have featured in surgical textbooks for very many years; yet comparatively recently the cases reaching the operating theatre of a hospital in one area in London were fewer than those dying without operation (James and Turner, 1951*). Somehow it should be possible to improve on this particular state of affairs. Rowbotham's monumental book, which has grown deservedly large in four editions during the past thirty years and which gives an excellent and comprehensive account of head injuries, is now perhaps too big to be read keenly by many who only occasionally have the care of cases of head injury. It is therefore to casualty officers, orthopaedic and general surgeons, general practitioners, and senior nurses, and not to neurosurgeons, that this book is addressed, in the hope that it is short enough to be thoroughly read and easily digested and that the index is sufficiently comprehensive.

No two cases of head injury are quite alike, so that controlled experiments for testing the superiority of one method of treat-

* *Lancet*, **2**, 45, 1951.

ment over another are virtually impossible. The true value of some courses of action that have been advocated is therefore difficult to assess, and this accounts for divergence of opinion about certain matters, usually of detail, in different neurosurgical centres. This is no new situation, as may be discovered by referring to Percivall Pott, writing on this very subject two centuries ago: "In matters of this sort positive proof and conviction are not in our power; all that we can do is, by making a comparison of the conduct and event of a number of similar cases, to come as near to truth as we can, and to get probability on our side." The aim of this book is to give a scheme which is essentially practical and as simple as possible, so that, for example, someone who is not particularly adept at lumbar puncture, or who finds this a disturbing procedure to himself and his patient, will know that it need not be done except under two clearly defined circumstances.

There are several aspects of head injuries to which little or no space is given: prevention is not considered relevant to the scope of this book, and details of certain operative procedures and radiological investigations and of other rather specialized techniques, such as hypothermia and controlled respiration, are not described, since they are at present the concern of those working in specialized units and in any case are appropriate only in a small minority of cases.

Most cases of head injury require a certain standard of *management* rather than active treatment; relatively few need the surgical operations which are so properly emphasized in textbooks. One difficulty is that all are potential candidates for such operations. That no head injury should be regarded lightly is soon learnt by all who do much accident work, and it is noteworthy that Pott started his book with the quotation of this same injunction from Hippocrates himself: "*nullum capitis vulnus contemnendum*".

The important task of assessment of a head injury takes place in the casualty department. In the planning of any accident service it is therefore essential to be sure that whoever has the initial responsibility for casualties is well versed in the necessary knowledge—or that someone who is so qualified is always available for consultation. Young anaesthetists who may have to deal with cases of combined head and other injury must be acquainted with the relationship between the respiratory system and the injured brain (pp. 6, 16, 21 and 34).

Reasons for the difficulty in organizing efficient head injury services throughout the country can be easily seen. Most serious cases are the result of high velocity road accidents and these tend to occur outside the towns and cities in which the more comprehensive hospitals containing neurosurgical units are situated. Therefore, accidents are usually taken to the nearest hospital, which may be a cottage hospital, and this generally has not facilities for the specialized care that a head injury requires. Despite difficulties, much good work is done under these circumstances by general and orthopaedic surgeons, but not infrequently they and general practitioners in the cottage hospitals are faced with the almost continuous anxiety that a severe case must incur.

A severe head injury is a disturbing factor in the efficient running of any ordinary hospital ward. Apart from the continuous need for careful nursing, the patient may be noisy, obstreperous, and a source of torment to other ill patients. Every hospital likely to admit such cases should be equipped with a sound-insulated side ward which will hold at least two patients. The importance of permitting a degree of noisiness and restlessness is considered in Chapter 3. At the Military Hospital for Head Injuries at Oxford, which was housed in St. Hugh's College during the last war, the library, being apart from the main wards, served a most useful purpose as the 'Noisy Boys' Ward'.

Severe head injuries, moreover, require extremely skilled care from nurses who should have had some special training in the problems of the unconscious patient. Such nurses cannot usually be conjured up at a moment's notice in a small hospital. People with these injuries should not therefore be taken to hospitals that have barely enough nurses to meet their ordinary commitments; special knowledge and quality in nursing care may be the deciding factor between the life and the death of a patient.

A patient with a head injury is a constant source of anxiety to those responsible for him. The intensity of observation that is necessary in the period immediately following the injury exceeds that required in almost any other condition. Even when one has the necessary knowledge and equipment for the performance of the various surgical measures required, it may be difficult, in doubtful or atypical cases, to know when and where, or whether to open the skull. Particular attention will be paid in this book to these matters.

To deal with head injuries requires a particular philosophy and a specially developed temperament. Those whose contemplation does not extend much beyond the purely mechanical aspects of an injury will find the subject difficult. Rapidly changing circumstances must be anticipated and met, and *to be one move ahead of the pathological process should always be the aim.* Without warning it may be necessary to control that most dangerous condition, status epilepticus, to diagnose meningitis promptly and then treat it energetically, or to localize and deal with intracranial haemorrhage without delay. One must also be able to understand patiently the psychological aspects of the patient's convalescence and the sequelae of his injury. Head injuries are in all ways most disruptive events, particularly to the peace of mind of anyone who is used to a relatively ordered clinical existence, and if this is governed by rules of thumb and fortified by restful nights, the impact is severe. It is understandable that head injuries are not popular with everyone.

Chapter 2

IN THE CASUALTY DEPARTMENT

Cerebral Concussion

It is unusual to witness the true state of cerebral concussion. In Britain the widely accepted definition of this condition is that of Wilfred Trotter, who held it to be "an essentially transient state due to head injury which is of instantaneous onset, manifests widespread symptoms of a purely paralytic kind, does not as such comprise any evidence of structural cerebral injury, and is always followed by amnesia for the actual moment of the accident" (that is to say, the accident *to the head*). This actual state is so transitory that it is seen only if the injury occurs in one's presence—in the street, say, or during a football game. The injured man may at first appear dead—pulseless and apnoeic—but recovery soon follows, and what one sees later are either the after-effects of concussion, or other complications of head injury. Rarely, death may occur in the early stages, owing to the inhalation of vomitus, particularly if the patient is also under the influence of alcohol, or, as experimental evidence suggests, because of failure of the respiratory centre to recover its function.

First Aid

Ensure Airway

As a first-aid measure it is therefore wise to ensure a good airway and to place the patient in an almost-prone position, if possible with the head lowered (Fig. 1), until the cough and swallowing reflexes have returned. If respiration has not started, *artificial respiration* should be given. Provided there is someone who can perform the procedure efficiently, there is much to be said for the immediate endotracheal intubation of all those who arrive in the accident room with cough and swallowing reflexes depressed. This allows the almost-prone position to be dispensed

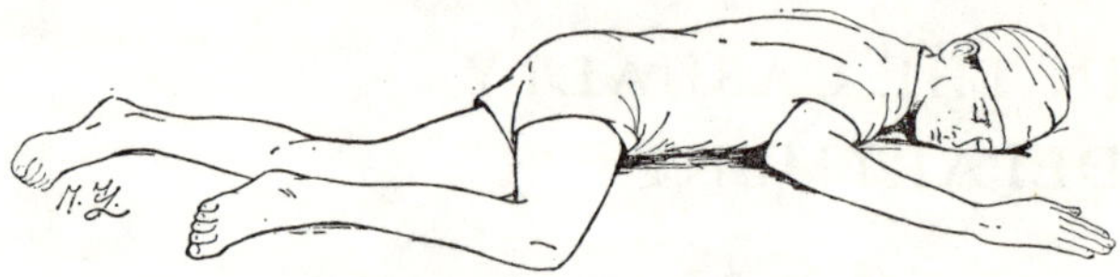

FIG. 1.—The almost-prone position. The uppermost arm and leg are flexed to provide stability.

with, enabling the patient to be examined safely and more easily; and it permits the trachea to be cleared by suction.

Haemorrhage

Any severe external haemorrhage should be the next concern. Usually a pad and firm (preferably crêpe) bandage will control a bleeding scalp wound adequately, but branches of the superficial temporal or occipital arteries may require individual attention. Much time can be wasted in trying to stop superficial bleeding; the best way to do this is to sew up the wound there and then. If a second pair of hands is available to compress the scalp against the skull, an inch or so from the wound margins, the operator's task will be greatly eased.

Shock

Surgical shock, if present, should be remedied without delay, and the head injury assessed subsequently. In such a case, the abdomen, chest, pelvis, and femora should be particularly examined for associated injuries because true shock—that is, peripheral circulatory failure—is rare in cases of head injury alone unless there has been severe haemorrhage. (See also p. 16).

Anoxia

Anoxia.—The brain is particularly vulnerable to anoxia (hypoxia) and may be exposed to it in several ways after injury. *Anoxic anoxia* may result from airway obstruction by the tongue, by laryngeal spasm or by the inhalation of blood, vomitus or secretions; from inadequate ventilation due to the injudicious administration of morphine; from associated pneumo- or haemothorax; or, later, from pneumonic consolidation, collapse or pulmonary oedema. *Anaemic anoxia* may occur from blood loss, particularly if the patient is already anaemic at the time of injury; and *stagnant anoxia* may accompany surgical shock.

These forms of anoxia may be present in powerful combination to threaten the already injured brain. By failing to provide the normal cough and swallowing reflexes, and by immobilizing the patient, the damaged brain may contribute very much to its own further destruction. To combat these dangers is within the power of any junior casualty officer who realizes that the provision of a free airway, the replacement of lost blood, and the maintenance of the systolic blood pressure above 100 mm. Hg. are urgent rather than routine matters.

It should always be remembered that, "Anoxaemia not only stops the machine, but wrecks the machinery."

PRELIMINARY ASSESSMENT OF THE HEAD INJURY

Question Witnesses

Detain for questioning anyone who comes with the patient; much valuable information may be obtained. At what time did the injury occur, and where? What was the patient's behaviour afterwards? Has he become more responsive since, or less? (Has there, in fact, been any kind of 'lucid interval'?) Was there any sort of convulsion? Ambulance men should always be interrogated, for they may give valuable information and may even have examined the pupils soon after the accident.

Careful Notes

All the information obtained should be scrupulously recorded in the notes, because it provides the earliest base-line from which it may be possible to tell, even at that early stage, that the patient's condition is already improving—or later, perhaps, that cerebral compression is in progress. For this reason, careful, concise and unambiguous notes are particularly important if several doctors are likely to be successively concerned with the care of the patient.

Record Times

The times of the accident, of the patient's admission, and of the first, and subsequent, clinical examinations should all be noted. These will greatly help any later observer to assess quickly how rapidly a patient's condition is worsening and to what extent there has been any 'lucid interval' between the initial concussion and deterioration of the level of responsiveness later, due to cerebral compression.

The Three Base-lines

You should then set about establishing base-lines from which you and others will have to work. The most important of these is the patient's level of responsiveness.

1. The Level of Responsiveness

Level of Responsiveness

Try to avoid indefinite terms, such as 'conscious', 'semi-coma' and 'stupor', whose meanings are not sufficiently precise. Is the patient alert or drowsy? Record what he will do. Will he answer questions rationally, or is he confused? Can he give his name and address? Is he correctly or reasonably orientated: does he know the day, the date and the year, and where he is? In assessing his responses, bear in mind the possibility that his speech functions may have been specifically damaged (dysphasia—see pp. 14 and 80).

Degrees of Responsiveness

If there is no response when his name is spoken, the patient should first be shouted at; then shaken gently; and, finally, stimulated uncomfortably by firm tickling of the axilla or scratching the soles of the feet. By his response to these graduated stimuli the level of 'consciousness' may be reasonably measured and recorded in terms that will be understood by anyone who may later be called upon to decide whether he is more, or less, responsive.

Amnesia

When he is fully rational and correctly orientated, *but not before*, you should estimate the length of time for which there has been loss of memory. With cerebral concussion there will, by definition, be loss of memory for the injury, and this will extend back in time for a variable but usually short period: this is the retrograde amnesia which is the hall-mark of cerebral concussion. For practical purposes, the duration of this amnesia is unimportant compared with that of the post-traumatic amnesia (P.T.A.) which follows. The length of the P.T.A. is useful knowledge. In the first place, it is a valuable index of the degree of cerebral injury, and it has the scientific merit that at least a rough degree of measurement is possible. Second, the period of absence from work shows some correlation with the duration of the P.T.A. when this amounts to more than about twenty-four hours. Finally, a late, retrospective assessment of the severity of a brain injury can be made many months after the injury if the P.T.A. is known.

'P.T.A.'

As in the earlier examination, it is better to put aside the more complicated problem of 'consciousness' and to consider how much the patient remembers. *The P.T.A. extends from the moment of injury to the time when continuous awareness and memory return.* The end-point may be difficult to determine and often some approximation must be accepted, but this matters little when a P.T.A. of "several days" is sufficient evidence of severity. In the great majority of cases it amounts to less than an hour, which indicates a relatively mild degree of concussion. Ask the patient where he was when he woke up and when his memory returned clearly and continuously. There may have been 'islands' of memory before continuous awareness was established, in which case they should be ignored. If there is still confusion of thought, estimates of amnesia are unreliable and the questioning should be deferred until the following day, when it will usually be found that the patient was still in the period of P.T.A. at the first interview and remembers nothing of it.

2. Abnormal Neurological Signs

C.N.S. Examination

The second base-line is that afforded by an examination of the functions of the central nervous system which is quite simple and is directed primarily towards those features which can be used to recognize a change in the patient's condition. Certain cranial nerve injuries may occur at the time of the injury and therefore cannot be used as indicators of any serious complication that may develop later. These should be noted at this stage, but they will be considered in more detail later, in Chapter 4. The important indicators with which we are now concerned are only two: the pupils, and cerebral hemisphere function.

The Pupils

(a) Pupillary Changes.—The importance of an ipsilateral dilating pupil as a sign of extradural haemorrhage is well known. Several points do, however, need to be stressed. First, an obvious one: that, unless the pupils have originally been observed to be equal and reacting, and *recorded as such*, the observation of inequality later may lead to confusion and even an unnecessary craniotomy. Hence the importance of the base-line. I have several times been called urgently to see cases where one fixed and dilated pupil has been present from the time of injury, or very soon after it, owing to a direct injury to the eye or orbit (traumatic mydriasis). With such an orbital injury it may in fact be the *optic* and not the oculomotor nerve that has been damaged, and this results in both pupils remaining immobile when the blind eye is illuminated, but reacting when the torch is shone in the opposite eye. It is a delayed paresis or complete paralysis of the pupillary constrictor fibres in the third cranial nerve (oculomotor nerve), regardless of which eye is

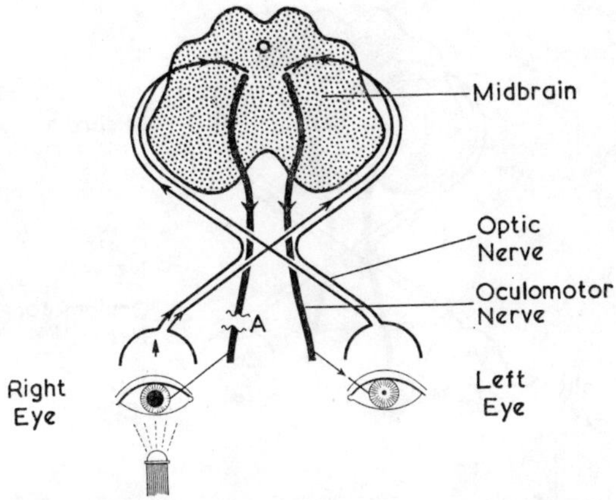

FIG. 2.—Right oculomotor (3rd) nerve lesion at A. Illumination of the right eye fails to constrict the pupil on that side (absent direct light reaction). On the left side the pupil constricts normally (consensual reaction present). Only the efferent (motor) pathway of the light reflex is interrupted, and only on the right side.

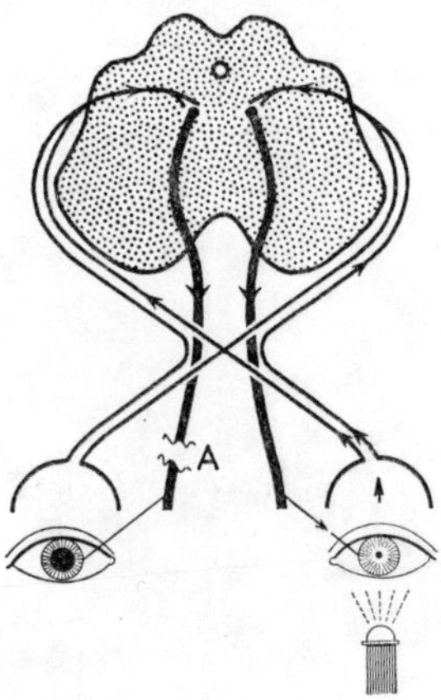

FIG. 3.—The same injury as in Fig. 2, but with the left eye illuminated. Each pupil reacts in the same way as in Fig. 2.

(The pupillary changes in Figs. 2 and 3 are those seen with an extradural haematoma on the right side.)

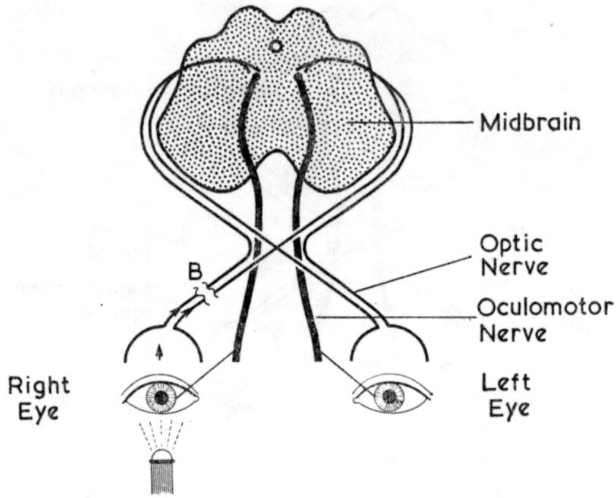

FIG. 4.—Right optic nerve injury at B. Illumination of the blind right eye fails to constrict either pupil because the afferent (sensory) pathway of the light reflex is interrupted early in its course at B (absent direct and consensual reactions).

FIG. 5.—The same injury as in Fig. 4, but with the left eye illuminated. There is no interruption at all of the light-reflex arcs, and both pupils therefore react (direct and consensual reactions present).

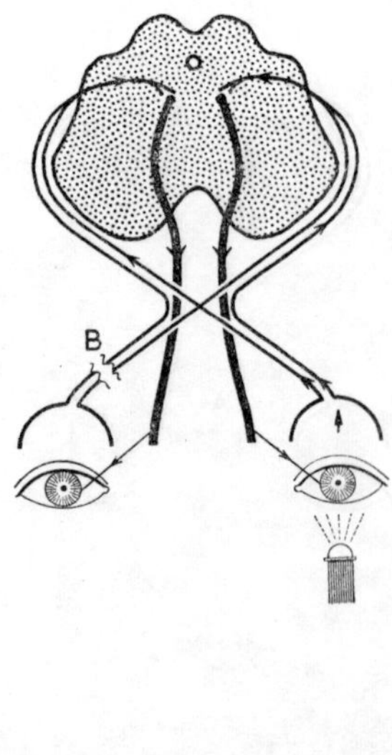

illuminated, that is of such importance in unilateral cerebral compression. These important alterations in the pupillary light reflex are illustrated by simplified diagrams in Figs. 2–5. *A bright torch should be used.*

Minor inequalities of the pupils may come and go and, in cases of doubt, re-examination at five-minute intervals should be carried out. It is important to examine the pupils properly before the eyes have become tightly closed through swelling of the lids, and after this has occurred, every possible effort must be made to see what is happening to them from time to time. Assistance may be required to restrain a restless patient and to help in opening the swollen and tender eyelids. The use of atropine, which dilates the pupils, should always be avoided at the early stage of a head injury.

Cerebral Hemisphere Dysfunction

(b) Signs of Increasing Cerebral Hemisphere Disturbance.—These may be an important indication, usually when taken in conjunction with a dilating pupil, that localized cerebral compression is in progress. An extradural haemorrhage over the motor regions of the frontal lobe will result in increasing weakness of the face and arm of the opposite side of the body (and, to a lesser extent usually, of the leg) which may occasionally be preceded or accompanied by an epileptic fit starting in these areas (Jacksonian epilepsy). The anoxic anoxia and cerebral venous congestion which accompanies the fit may lead to a rapid worsening in the patient's condition.

The recognition of lateralized weakness in a patient who is not co-operative requires only a little practice. If the patient is restless, the relative amount of movement of each side can be observed. Bilateral supra-orbital pressure will cause grimacing which will show whether there is facial weakness; the arms should then be lifted and released and any falling away of one of them noted, and the legs may be tested in a similar manner. The response to painful stimuli applied to each limb should be seen, and any increase in tone sought. Finally, the tendon reflexes may be tested, but these, the most conventionally observed functions, usually provide such a delicate indication of any minor contusion of the pyramidal tracts that their usefulness is limited. Thus, it is common for any case of moderately severe head injury to show discrepancy in the reflexes of the two sides in the early stages, and one or both plantar responses are frequently extensor (Babinski) in type.

Signs of disturbed cortical sensory function are not so easily elicited in these patients, owing to insufficient co-operation, but when demonstrable the presence of a 'homonymous' hemianopia is an important localizing sign; if this develops subsequent to the initial examination an intracerebral clot (in the brain on the side opposite to the visual field defect) rather than an extracerebral one is likely to be present, because the optic radiations are less liable to be disturbed by the more diffuse compression of a clot over the surface of the brain (Fig. 6).

Dysphasia

If the clot is forming over the left (dominant) cerebral hemisphere, particularly in the area where the frontal, temporal and parietal lobes meet, right-handed persons will develop some loss of the faculty of speech (dysphasia), and this may be recognized if they are still sufficiently alert. A sensitive test is to confront the patient with a series of ten or so common objects, and to ask him to name them. If dysphasic he will be unable to do this, to an extent that is clearly abnormal. If worse affected, he will be unable to converse lucidly and may have difficulty in understanding people who are speaking to him, or what he reads.

'Decerebrate rigidity' of the 'physiological' extensor muscles of the limbs is commonly present in various degrees following a severe brain injury and, although consistent with recovery, should suggest a particularly guarded prognosis as to the degree of recovery. The spasms may be intermittent and associated with periods of increased respiratory activity and may occur spontaneously or in response to a stimulus.

3. Other Vital Functions

Pulse, B.P., and Respiration

This term will be used to cover the pulse rate, arterial pressure and respiratory rate, which together make up the third of the base-lines. Typically, a progressive slowing of the pulse rate, a progressive rise

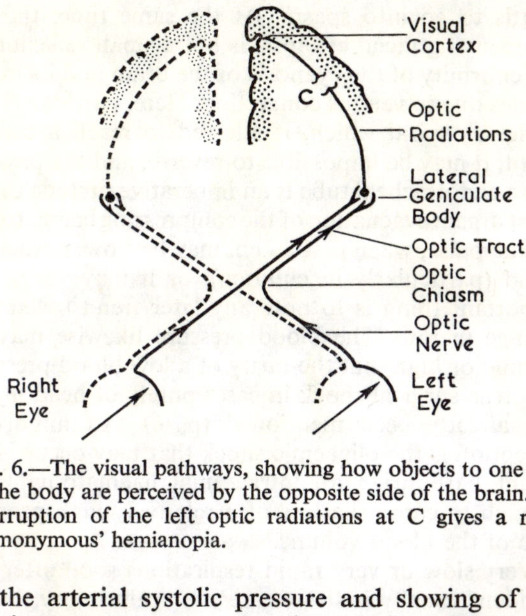

FIG. 6.—The visual pathways, showing how objects to one side of the body are perceived by the opposite side of the brain. An interruption of the left optic radiations at C gives a right 'homonymous' hemianopia.

in the arterial systolic pressure and slowing of the respiratory rate are concomitants of cerebral compression. Of these, the slowing pulse is usually the earliest sign, whilst extreme slowing of respiration comes late and is an urgent warning that periodic breathing, which may or may not be of the classical Cheyne-Stokes type, is likely soon to follow, with total apnoea and death in its wake. By this time, a rapid rise in the pulse rate may have occurred, together with a fall in the blood pressure, whose compensatory elevation can no longer be maintained in order to supply the compressed brain with blood. Here it should be stressed, however, that this terminal sequence of events may never be reached, owing to the occurrence of cardiac arrest from *asphyxia*. This can occur when respiration is still fairly rapid, but noisy and stertorous, because the disturbance of bulbar function allows both the tongue to fall back and the glottis to go into spasm. At the same time, the accompanying facial cyanosis is but a small reflexion of the enormity of the cyanosis of the brain and its membranes due to venous congestion. Here, particularly, is a vicious spiral which, if allowed to reach a certain point, it may be impossible to reverse, and the passage of an endotracheal tube is an imperative prelude to the most urgent evacuation of the compressing haematoma.

The pulse, when first taken, may be slow, normal or rapid (particularly in children), or it may vary. The important thing is to note any later trend towards a change in rate. The blood pressure likewise may be normal or high, but the rarity of a low blood pressure and true surgical shock in cases purely of head injury has already been mentioned (p. 6). An important exception is the oligaemic shock that may occur in an infant harbouring an intracranial haematoma large enough to cause the loss of a relatively high proportion of the blood volume.

Very slow or very rapid respirations soon after the accident usually indicate a severe brain injury, but it must be ascertained that the tachypnoea is not the result of injury within the thorax, and that slow breathing is not due to morphine having been administered. Periodic breathing also suggests a serious injury, but not, as is commonly supposed, necessarily an irrecoverable one.

Temperature

The temperature may be subnormal, particularly if

there is shock. If the serious complication of hyperpyrexia occurs, it is often later; this is considered in the next chapter (pp. 35–36).

Papilloedema

Although acute papilloedema and retinal haemorrhages may be seen immediately after a severe head injury, swelling of the optic disks does not necessarily develop later as a sign of increased intracranial pressure resulting from an extra- or sub-dural haematoma. However, a patient whose recovery appears otherwise to be proceeding perfectly satisfactorily may be discovered to have marked papilloedema when examined routinely a week or two after injury. Such an occurrence always warrants neurosurgical investigation, though the condition may prove to be a benign form of intracranial hypertension (communicating hydrocephalus) which recovers spontaneously. This complication may also produce lateral rectus weakness, especially in children (see also p. 68).

Blood or C.S.F. from the Nose and Ears

Bleeding from the nose is *per se* of little importance; it may indicate a fracture of the anterior cranial fossa, but more often it follows local damage to the nose. Bleeding from an ear, however, is usually evidence of a fracture of the petrous bone. Otoscopy is then fruitless and risks the introduction of infection; the ear is probably best left alone in the acute stage. But occasionally the ear drum is not ruptured and blood remains confined to the middle ear; otoscopy under these circumstances is perfectly safe and will disclose a blue, bulging drum. A day or two later a bruise may appear over the mastoid process (Battle's sign), a further indication of fracture (see also p. 21).

Fractured Petrous Bone

Otoscopy

Leakage of cerebrospinal fluid, from the nose (rhinorrhoea) or, more rarely, from the ear (otorrhoea) is of greater importance and should alert one to the possibility that meningitis may occur. The management of these complications is discussed on pages 59–63.

Meningism

It is appropriate to introduce at this stage a not infrequent but somewhat neglected accompaniment of head injury. *Traumatic subarachnoid haemorrhage* and the meningeal inflammation that it produces may be the cause of much headache and irritability (the so-called 'cerebral irritation'), and perhaps of some of the other symptoms which persist after what may have been a relatively mild head injury. Bloodstained cerebrospinal fluid (c.s.f.) may be found after apparently mild 'cerebral concussion', such that a ruptured cerebral aneurysm or angiomatous malformation may even be suspected (and occasionally found). It is usually unnecessary, however, and wrong at this early stage, to resort to lumbar puncture in order to diagnose this complication, for it will be revealed clinically *if the patient's neck is tested for stiffness on anteflexion* and Kernig's sign also sought. These examinations, which should always be included in a case of head injury, are usually omitted, while valuable time is wasted with deliberations over the more familiar signs, such as that of Babinski, which in itself is of little practical importance.

Test for Neck Stiffness and Kernig's Sign

Having emphasized this point, a qualification must now be made, which is that the signs of meningism usually take some hours to develop fully and may not be much in evidence in the casualty department. Minor degrees should be sought, however, but the examination must be repeated in the ward the next day, when quite marked neck stiffness and Kernig's sign may be present and the patient has regained consciousness sufficiently to complain of headache and perhaps admit to photophobia. If there is also fever and any suspicion of bacterial meningitis, then lumbar puncture should be performed without delay (see also

Test again the next day

pp. 40 and 61). Traumatic subarachnoid haemorrhage may be the cause of considerable and justifiable vexation to a patient who is sent home from the casualty department after an apparently mild and uncomplicated concussion only to awake the following morning feeling really ill. *Purely neurological signs of abnormality are absent and there may not be a skull fracture.* If the patient is told to get up and resume normal activity as soon as possible, the stage may be set for a period of apparent neurosis for which there is in fact a perfectly sound organic basis, added to which there may be an understandable resentment that such harsh advice should have been given.

Neck Injuries

Degrees of neck stiffness may, for the purposes of record and assessing progress, be conveniently measured by the number of fingers' breadths from the chin to the suprasternal notch when the head is anteflexed to the point of discomfort. Bony injuries of the neck must of course be distinguished from meningism: local tenderness should be sought and restriction and pain on movements other than anteflexion. Soft-tissue injuries of the neck are not uncommonly associated with head injuries, particularly those of the occipital region, and may be a cause of headache and difficulty in differential diagnosis. The presence or absence of Kernig's sign will, however, be of assistance, and in all cases of doubt the cervical spine should be x-rayed, when pre-existing cervical spondylosis may be revealed.

Differential Diagnosis of Head Injury

Sometimes it is not certain whether there has in fact been a head injury. An epileptic fit may have passed unobserved or unrecognized, and the patient is admitted, say from the street, in the post-ictal state. A spontaneous subarachnoid haemorrhage may have occurred in a relatively young person under equivocal

Examine carefully for External Evidence of Head Injury

circumstances. An old lady, living alone, may be found at the bottom of her stairs unconscious, having had a stroke. Provided there is external evidence or x-ray evidence of a head injury and *whatever the actual cause of the injury, she must be managed as a case of head injury, for she is just as liable to all the complications*. This cannot be stressed too strongly; it does not matter whether the cause of the fall was a medical condition ("hypertension: ? stroke"), a neurological one ("a known epileptic"), or an ear-nose-and-throat one ("Ménière's disease"); the primary condition is not for the time being usually the important one. Administrative niceties, concerning the specialty under which the case should be admitted, can be observed later—perhaps after an extradural clot has been evacuated. For the time being the case is one of a head injury.

Drug Coma

Coma resulting from an overdose of barbiturate drugs is not often associated with a head injury; it is a tranquil form of unconsciousness. In morphine overdosage, the pupils are of course constricted; and with atropine or hyoscine (a rare cause nowadays) the pupils are dilated and the patient's skin is usually flushed and dry. Diabetic and insulin coma should be easily recognizable.

Alcohol

By contrast, alcohol and head injury are frequently in combination, especially in the busier and wilder parts of our cities where the large general hospitals are often situated. It is tempting not to admit a patient who has clearly been drinking and whose confusional state is thought to be entirely the result of the alcohol rather than the bruise on the head which might, after all, have been an effect of quite a trivial blow. This temptation should, whenever possible, be firmly resisted. A retrospective assessment is much safer. Here is a case of Percivall Pott's (although, admittedly, one in which the correct course of action was pretty clear): "A Drayman, drunk and sleeping, fell from his dray. . . . He was brought to hospital senseless . . . the next day the man was so well and so perfectly the master of what sense he had, that I was inclined to believe that a great deal of last night's appearance was owing principally to liquor."

The scalp should be most carefully searched for small cuts, abrasions and contusions. Localized oedema of the scalp, as distinct from a contusion, should also be sought; this may occur over a fracture and frequently becomes progressively pronounced if an extradural haemorrhage is occurring deep to the fracture. In this, it resembles the now rare 'Pott's puffy tumour', which appears over the site of an extradural abscess. Sometimes no external injury is found, but concussion may have occurred none the less, and occasionally a subdural haematoma will follow.

Localized Scalp Oedema

The cause of any unexplained fall should be carefully considered. Healthy, sober people do not normally 'just fall down' with sufficient clumsiness to damage the head. In the very young and in the elderly, however, gait may be ataxic and the postural reflexes inefficient. But alcohol remains the common cause of impairment of locomotion and judgement in adults. Minor forms of epilepsy may also pass unrecognized until a series of admissions to the casualty department leads to diagnosis.

Why did they Fall?

Other Injuries

During the course of the neurological examination the opportunity should be taken to examine the rest of the body for associated injuries. Once again the danger of attributing surgical shock purely to the head injury must be stressed: abdominal or chest injuries should be sought and, if severe, they ought usually to be given priority in treatment, since the stagnant anoxia of shock itself may have a most adverse effect on the injured brain, as will any anoxic anoxia that may result from a chest injury.

Shock

In most cases, however, the head injury will be the greater potential danger to life itself, but a careful assessment of the combination of injuries must be made in each case. A compound limb fracture, for example, will need early attention, usually under general anaesthesia. There should be close co-operation between all concerned so that all the various aspects of treatment can be properly timed and co-ordinated. The head injury should be re-assessed immediately before the induction of anaesthesia and afterwards, in case signs of cerebral compression should occur during this period; the anaesthetic itself should be as light and as short as is feasible, in order that these signs should not be obscured. Premedication with drugs which depress consciousness or affect the pupils should be avoided. A clear airway will of course be vital, and any straining or venous congestion avoided completely. There is every reason to keep on emphasizing these points, because most young anaesthetists who are called to these cases at night have little or no experience of these particular difficulties.

Compound Limb Fractures

General Anaesthesia

One case may be cited as an example of the degree of alertness that is required on the part of all concerned. A ruptured spleen occurred in combination with a head injury. After the spleen had been removed, the anaesthetist noticed that one pupil, which had been normal at the time of induction, was larger and more sluggish than the other. The prompt removal of an extradural haematoma then saved the patient's life for the second time within an hour, and this might not have been possible had the pupillary reflexes been masked by drugs or by an unnecessary depth of anaesthesia, or if the anaesthetist had been less vigilant.

Avoid General Anaesthesia if possible

It is a sound rule that *general anaesthesia should be avoided if possible* in the early stages of any but the mildest head injuries. A second rule is that a patient who is insufficiently conscious to require general anaesthesia is sufficiently unconscious to need an anaesthetist or someone who can assure a safe airway throughout the operation.

Maxillo-facial Injuries

The combination of a head injury and a maxillo-facial injury calls for specialized co-operation which is usually available only in the larger hospital centres. The two most important considerations are the maintenance of a free airway, and the recognition of fracturing of the frontal, ethmoidal or sphenoidal air sinuses which may result in c.s.f. rhinorrhoea and/or meningitis. Definitive treatment of jaw fractures (which are not themselves a danger to life) should usually be delayed if the brain injury is a severe one, but a maxillo-facial surgeon should be consulted as early as possible and the course of action decided.

Skull X-rays

Not long ago there was a mistaken notion that the skull need be x-rayed only for the medico-legal purpose of establishing whether or not a fracture was present. This at least recognized the relative unimportance of skull fractures in themselves, but the reason given is the very last one which should be entertained. Good x-rays should be taken soon after injury whenever possible—the postero-anterior, the 30° antero-posterior (Towne's) and the lateral views being the usual ones. But it must always be considered whether an ill, restless patient is fit to travel, some distance maybe, to the X-ray Department, there to be moved on and off the table, and dealt with by perhaps a junior and inexperienced radiographer in the middle of the night—and whether the resulting pictures will be worthwhile. Portable skull x-rays are only occasionally better than none at all, but sometimes even a cockeyed film will show a depressed fracture that may escape detection in a properly aligned view, so that *all films that are taken should be preserved.*

Why is it a good practice to take x-rays if possible soon after an injury at night, and not the next morning when conditions may be much more favourable? Intelligent anticipation is a most important part of head-injury work, and anything which suggests that one should watch for a particular complication is worth having. It is good, therefore, to know as early as possible whether there is fracturing of the air sinuses, or intracranial air, which might result in meningitis (pp. 61, 63 and 83); or whether a fracture line crosses the middle meningeal artery, *and on which side*, for extradural haemorrhage without a fracture is uncommon in adults, although less so in children. It is also better that the presence and extent of a compound depressed fracture should be accurately seen on the x-rays than inadequately felt by probing around the wound in the casualty department.

Pineal Shift

The lateral projection should be examined for the presence of pineal calcification which, if present, should then be sought in the antero-posterior views. These latter views should be perfectly true, in which case a pineal shift of more than 2.0 mm. is usually significant. But if they are not straight, there may be the false impression that the pineal is displaced.

Echo-Encephalography

An initial belief that, in the Echo-E.G., here at last was an answer to the casualty officer's prayer, has not been sustained. But *for someone who has already acquired the basic knowledge* that the earlier sections of this book seek to impart, a reliable modern machine will provide a useful extension to the unaided senses. But the user must have been shown how to use it properly, and be prepared to employ it frequently in order that practice will make him thoroughly familiar with the various tricks that it may play on the untutored and inexperienced.

Its advantage is that the method may quickly and

painlessly—and in the casualty department—reveal a shift of the midline structures of the brain. But if a displaced pineal body has already indicated this on x-ray, the Echo-E.G. is superfluous and valuable time should not be wasted when there is sufficient clinical evidence of an extradural haematoma.

The Wound

Unless haemorrhage has called for earlier attention, it is proper that the wound itself should be left until the preceding matters have been considered. Appropriate measures should be taken against tetanus, and the proper wound toilet that follows is probably most important in making cephalic tetanus now extremely rare in this country.

Shaving

The hair should be clipped and then *shaved for at least two inches all around the wound* after the area has been well soaped. If a sharp razor is not available, a large scalpel blade of the Bard-Parker type will suffice. After this has been done, the wound will often look much less formidable and may be more thoroughly cleaned. Puncture-wounds should be particularly sought and recognized, and the possibility of skull penetration always borne in mind.

Has there been Penetration?

If, because of the patient's general condition, or for any other reason, it is desired to postpone the excision and suture, it is reasonably safe to do so; for it was shown during World War II that the incidence of infection increased only slightly if the wound was not dealt with until between twelve and eighteen hours after it had been received. But the wound should be covered with a sterile dressing and not exposed to hospital organisms.

The operation itself should be done in a theatre if possible. After cleaning the wound and draping, a local analgesic is injected around the margins into the scalp tissues *superficial to the aponeurotic layer*, where the nerves and blood vessels lie, and not into the sub-

Local Analgesia

aponeurotic space where it is ineffective. Lignocaine (Xylocaine), 1 per cent with adrenaline, 1:250,000, produces both good analgesia and vasoconstriction.

If the wound is a clean-cut one and the margins healthy and bleeding, no excision is necessary; but if it is dirty, ragged or contused it is better to cut out the whole wound cleanly down to the pericranium, *after first testing that the mobility of the scalp, which varies very considerably, will allow the edges to come together afterwards—this should be done before the local anaesthetic is injected.* If the aponeurosis has been split, the wound will gape, and it is better sutured in two layers, the deeper inverted stitches approximating the strong avascular aponeurosis under whatever tension is required, and those in the skin serving merely to bring together the edges without tension or embarrassment to the blood supply. For the buried sutures there is nothing better than waxed silk (e.g., Mersilk, size 3/0). A mere split in the skin superficial to the aponeurosis requires only a single layer of stitches.

Plastic Surgery

For the technique of closing larger gaps in the scalp, readers should refer to the plastic surgical methods described in a short, lucid paper by the late Sir Harold Gillies.*

Wound Infection

The scalp, by virtue of its generous blood supply, is usually most tolerant of careless and shoddy stitching, but it should be remembered that, unlike most infected wounds elsewhere, a scalp infection is potentially more dangerous and its outcome may prove fatal. When a scalp wound does become infected, it is usually the result of inefficient or too long-delayed excision and suture.

Admission to Hospital

The next stage of the patient's management will usually take place in the hospital ward, but no formalities of admission should stop him being taken

* *Lancet,* **2,** 310, 1944.

directly to the operating theatre in his outdoor clothes should evidence of developing cerebral compression have already been established, for minutes may count. Burr-holes have been successfully made, without asepsis, even before the theatre could be reached, when rapid failure of respiration has demanded that this should be done.

Which cases of head injury should be admitted to hospital? Unfortunately, expediency, usually owing to shortage of beds, frequently dictates that many of the apparently milder cases are sent home, and these will inevitably include some patients who have sustained traumatic subarachnoid haemorrhage and a few who will develop other forms of intracranial haemorrhage or complications. Practices differ, but, ideally, patients in the following categories should be admitted at least overnight:

(1) All who have retrograde amnesia.
(2) Those with skull fractures.
(3) Those showing undue headache, vomiting or other unexplained or worrying symptoms.
(4) All children brought to hospital after a head injury. They are more difficult to assess than adults. Hydrocephalic children may react particularly severely to quite mild injuries.

The aphorism of Hippocrates, quoted in the introduction, should always be remembered: no head injury, *however trivial*, should be regarded lightly.

Chapter 3

IN THE WARD

The Principle of Retrospective Diagnosis

An accurate diagnosis of the complexity of a head injury is not usually possible in the early stages. A linear fracture of the right parietal bone may be seen on the x-rays, but to diagnose the patient's condition thus is to ignore the unimportance of such a fracture in itself. A bad mistake is to diagnose simply cerebral concussion in the accident room and to have to operate later the same night to evacuate an extradural clot which was accumulating at the time of the initial diagnosis. The danger of diagnosing a relatively minor aspect of the head injury is that this will be the official and accepted diagnosis with which the patient enters the ward; and those looking after him, especially if they are inexperienced, may be lulled into the mistaken belief that there is nothing more to be said; for is not concussion benign and reversible, and are not linear skull fractures unimportant? An entirely wrong psychological attitude may be encouraged instead of an alert, watchful one in which nothing is taken for granted. It is much better simply to label all cases **Head Injury** initially, and to fractionize the diagnosis *in retrospect* at the time of the patient's discharge: e.g.,

1. Cerebral concussion
2. Traumatic subarachnoid haemorrhage
3. Simple linear right parietal fracture
4. Multiple scalp lacerations; etc.

The Severely Injured

We will first consider the patient who is still unconscious when he reaches the ward and who may remain in this state for several days. He is in a minority group, but his condition is precarious and his management most important.

Observation of the Unconscious Patient

Continuous Observation

In the ward, a process of continuous observation is immediately started and is carried on without interruption, the ward staff establishing their own baselines without delay and both the doctor and the nurses being thereby able to decide at any time later whether the patient is *better*, *worse*, or *the same*.

Nurses' Responsibility

The nurses' particular concern will be with the degree of responsiveness and with the recording of this, the pulse and respiration rates, the blood pressure (the systolic being usually sufficient) and temperature. These should be measured at least half-hourly during the first twelve hours and afterwards until full consciousness is regained, and charted together with a brief description of the level of responsiveness and a note of the relative size and reactions of the pupils. (A specimen chart is given as Appendix 3.)

Charting

Charts should not be too elaborate; if they are, there is a danger that, in the eagerness to fill them in accurately, their objective may be lost sight of and the significance of a changing picture missed. This may appear to be a paradoxical statement, but I have several times experienced this very danger in cases of extradural haemorrhage where the general trend of events had been very clear on the chart for some time before its importance was appreciated. For this reason, I do not favour the routine drawing, in addition to the examining of pupillary size by the nursing staff. The nurse has quite enough to do already and *if there is any change in the pupils worthy of record, a doctor should be informed.* It is an irrelevance to note on a chart the fluctuation in size of both pupils equally, which occurs commonly; but any change towards inequality should be an alerting signal. Minor inequalities may, however, come and go and, if they are re-examined in five minutes, the pupils may have become equal once again. If not, and particularly if the discrepancy is more marked, the doctor should be summoned immediately. Unnecessary calls are bound to be made, but there is no better occasion for being safe rather than sorry. When the eyelids are swollen it may be difficult to examine the pupils regularly, but assistance in holding open the lids must be obtained in order that this important observation can be made.

(a) General Care of the Unconscious Patient

Once in bed, the unconscious patient should be placed almost prone and with the head slightly lowered so that the airway is clear (Fig. 1). If blinking and the corneal reflexes are absent, care must be taken that the cornea does not rub against the pillow, towel or bedclothes beneath the head, particularly if the eyes remain open. Regular irrigation or lubrication of the eyes in such cases will prevent the glazing or frank ulceration of the cornea which may develop and which may, if allowed to go unchecked, then necessitate more active measures, even tarsorrhaphy. A simple precaution, useful when eye-closure is slow to return, is to keep the eye shut by means of a single stitch through the loose skin at the centre of the upper lid only, just above the lashes. The ends of the stitch are left long enough to be secured to the cheek with a small piece of strapping and are released whenever the eye needs to be examined or irrigated.

Care of the Eyes

Avoid Sedative Drugs

Sedative drugs should be avoided completely at this stage. The most important reason for this is that the assessment of the level of responsiveness due to the injury becomes more difficult or impossible when the patient is under the influence also of depressant drugs which may moreover act capriciously on the injured brain. Secondly, a certain amount of restlessness is beneficial from the point of view of the chest and for the relief from any prolonged pressure on the skin over prominent bony points where sores might develop —the nurses are, in fact, saved the regular turning that would be needed were the patient to be lying quiet and still. Similarly, a noisy patient expands his lungs in a way that no physiotherapist can expect to do artificially. Noise can of course be a great annoyance to other patients and to the nursing staff, particularly at night, but this nuisance could be mitigated by the use of sound-insulation. Every hospital which receives an appreciable number of head injury cases should have a sound-insulated cubicle capable of holding two beds and with a double-glazed window through which the patient may be easily observed.

Restlessness

Noisiness

Sound Insulation

An over-restless patient may require some form of physical restraint (however objectionable this may be to those who are conscious of the relaxations now being practised in mental hospitals). It is the patient's welfare that must be considered, and his relatives, if properly counselled, are usually the last to make any objection. The wrists, and the ankles if necessary, may be encircled with adhesive orthopaedic felt over which a bandage may be tied with a clove-hitch and secured to the sides of the bed. Specially constructed leather thongs are also available. The patient is thus prevented from pulling out a gastric tube and from placing faecally contaminated fingers in a scalp wound. The wound should always be protected with a dressing and not, in the fashion sometimes for wounds elsewhere, left exposed or sprayed with some plastic preparation. There is all the difference between a patient with, say, a superficial arm wound who is

Physical Restraint

Dressings

mentally normal and one with a scalp wound who is confused and whose roving fingers might be to blame for death from intracranial sepsis.

Falling out of Bed

Next, the patient must be guarded, as far as is possible, from a fall from the bed. To have him on a mattress on the floor is one answer to the problem, but nursing is difficult and the method encounters aesthetic objections. Detachable bed-sides are not entirely satisfactory because, if the patient succeeds in surmounting them, he has further to fall. A net over the top of the bed and its sides is usually effective, but this too will offend those whose deference to a more humanitarian attitude towards mentally disturbed patients obscures the important need of the patient for protection from further injury. As it is, the number of patients who fall out of hospital beds every day must be enormous.

Distended Bladder

It must be remembered that the discomfort of a distended bladder is a potent cause of restlessness in a stuporous patient, and this should always be sought and remedied; the tranquillity that ensues is often dramatic.

Bedsores

The Skin.—Attention to the skin should of course be unremitting from the start, and with good, informed nursing (and enough nurses) bedsores should hardly ever appear. This is where much of the nurses' hard work comes: regular turning of the patient from side to side (the most important single measure); cleaning with soap and water and then light, gentle massage with Vaseline or barrier-cream over pressure-points, particularly if there is any reddening; and local protection of any areas where the viability of the skin appears to be in real jeopardy by encircling the affected point with a wide ring of orthopaedic felt in the manner of a corn plaster. Prevention here is everything: once started, a bedsore may take a very long time to heal.

(b) Special Care of the Unconscious Patient

In the past many patients died in hospital after a serious head injury as a result of the *complications* of unconsciousness itself rather than directly from brain damage, intracranial haemorrhage or sepsis. The greatest advance in the treatment of head injuries in recent years has come from the recognition of the ill-effects of coma and from their energetic prevention and treatment. The account that follows is applicable to many patients who are in deep coma from any cause. It is the nursing staff who carry out the major part of the treatment, and therefore if head injuries are to be well treated there must be a generous allocation of nurses for this purpose.

The Respiratory Passages.—If the coughing and swallowing reflexes are depressed, and particularly if they are absent, continuous vigilance will be required in order to maintain an adequate passage of air to the lungs. Blood and vomitus are both liable to enter the lungs. A severe brain injury is frequently associated with an excess of secretions from both the air passages and the salivary glands, and it is important to realize that fluid is accumulating primarily in the mouth as well as lower down towards the lungs. *The patient's head should be lowered and he should be almost prone* so that drainage is towards the open mouth (Fig. 1).

Head-down and almost prone

Suction Machine

An efficient suction machine is essential. This is connected to a soft plastic catheter which should be moistened and passed gently through the mouth or, sometimes with greater effect, through a nostril; it should be large enough to remove viscid mucus, blood clot and vomitus. If the patient coughs in response to the stimulus of the catheter in the pharynx or trachea, so much the better; for the lungs will then discharge otherwise inaccessible material, which is sucked away. It is a mistake to administer atropine with the object of diminishing secretions: it merely makes them more tenacious and difficult to extract. If a more viscid secretion does occur, a steam tent may be beneficial. Penicillin (0.5 mega-units twice daily) is probably wise prophylaxis under these circumstances.

Physiotherapy, in the form of measures such as pummelling the chest, may be useful, and the important objective is to produce coughing. This sort of activity is best combined with energetic suction when the patient is turned from one side to the other every two to four hours; it can be done by the nursing staff if no physiotherapist is available. These measures (or the permission of some restlessness and noisiness) will do much to diminish the complications of inhalation pneumonia and collapse of the lung, and hence anoxia of the injured brain (p. 6).

Tracheostomy and Intubation

Tracheostomy.—Tracheostomy is no longer a routine procedure for cases of severe head injury. This discrimination is welcome because it is an operation with complications: notably, infection, but also a blocked or coughed-out single tube, haemorrhage, pneumothorax and mediastinitis, which have all been reported and have themselves led to death. The important thing is that *the operation should be properly performed.* It is unnecessary to carry out emergency tracheostomy under adverse operating conditions when endotracheal intubation will serve the same purpose. The tube's inflatable cuff should be let down

Indications

for a few minutes every two hours. If after forty-eight hours, it appears that the airway will still require support, then tracheostomy should be performed as a formal operation. Other candidates for tracheostomy will be those known to suffer already from chronic bronchitis or bronchiectasis. An incompletely conscious patient with a bilaterally fractured mandible who shows no signs of early recovery should have the operation promptly.

At all times the great influence of respiratory function

over the damaged brain should be borne in mind. Blood-gas estimations may be utilized to identify and correct any deviations from the normal.

Tracheostomy Tubes

During the first few days, the tracheostomy tube should be a cuffed one, which when inflated will prevent blood, vomitus and secretions from entering the bronchi. Again, the cuff should be released every two hours. Later, a less irritating tube is substituted and the silver ones, such as Durham's, are probably still the best. They have the added safety of an inner tube, if this is left free to be coughed out should it become obstructed. Humidification of the inspired air is desirable.

Humidification

Infection

It is useful to know in advance what organisms are colonizing a tracheostomy in case they should give rise to frank infection, when the appropriate antibiotic can be given promptly. Swabs may therefore be taken from the tube once or twice a week, but the mere presence of organisms is no warrant for the use of antibiotics in the absence of fever and clinical signs of lung infection.

'Ribena' Test

Before removing a tracheostomy tube it is as well to test the efficiency of the swallowing mechanism. Blackcurrant juice (Ribena) may be given by mouth and then looked for in aspirated tracheal secretions. Gastric and oesophageal reflux into the trachea may be similarly detected where feeding is through a gastric tube.

Hyperpyrexia.—Damage to the thermostatic mechanism in the hypothalamus may result in a dangerous and *even a lethal* degree of fever which must be carefully watched for and promptly prevented. The brain appears to be especially sensitive to high temperature—and in these patients it is already a damaged brain. There may be a delay of twelve hours or more after injury before hyperpyrexia occurs and it seems to come particularly at night. At one moment the thermometer may read 38°C. (100°F.) and half an hour later

40°C. (105°F.) or more. It is wise not to allow the temperature to rise above 38.5°C. (101°F.), and readings at this stage should be taken rectally; this is a more accurate method, and may show values considerably higher than those obtained from the mouth or axilla. The temperature should be taken at ten- or fifteen-minute intervals during these times of crisis. Meanwhile, the bedclothes should be removed and the patient sponged with cold water. Ice (which should be readily available) in bags should be applied to the naked body, or a sheet may be wetted with ice-cold water, laid over the naked patient, and electric fans, with rubber vanes, turned on him so that he is rapidly cooled by evaporation, in the fashion of a butter cooler. It is almost always possible to reduce the temperature well below 38.5°C. (101°F.), *where it should be maintained*, if necessary with the aid of chlorpromazine, 25 or 50 mg. six-hourly, given preferably by mouth or tube, but if necessary intramuscularly. This lowering of the temperature towards normal should not be confused with *induced hypothermia*. 'Deep freezing' appears now to have only a very limited application to the management of severe head injury. The important thing that anyone can do is to maintain so far as possible a temperature near to normal in the face of a tendency for it to rise to exceptional and dangerous heights.

Rectal Temperature

Differential Diagnosis of Pyrexia

Needless to say, other causes of pyrexia—chest, urinary or wound infection and meningitis—should be thought of and excluded before the high temperature itself is treated.

Fluid Balance.—Few neurosurgeons nowadays restrict the fluid intake in cases of head injury in the belief that they are dehydrating a waterlogged brain with benefit to the patient. It is now generally felt that it is better to give adequate fluid than to withhold it, though there is no great hurry to start. About twenty hours after the injury, the tendency to vomit will have receded, the gut will be more receptive and the phase of water-retention will be finishing. If the patient will not swallow, a gastric tube should be passed through the nose, any stomach fluid aspirated, and 30 ml. tap water instilled hourly. If after four hours this quantity is being absorbed, 60 ml. glucose-water may be given as a 10 per cent solution (50 grammes glucose per pint of tap water) every hour, aspiration of the tube confirming each time that there is no fluid accumulating in the stomach. If all is well after a further twelve hours, the quantity is increased to 90 ml. hourly, and twelve hours later the diet can be strengthened to the same quantity of half-strength milk.

Water and Electrolyte Balance

If much water is being lost through vomiting, in respiratory and salivary secretions, as profuse c.s.f. rhinorrhoea or through sweating during hyperpyrexia, the intake of fluid must be correspondingly increased. A satisfactory output of urine should be obtained and always measured if possible. On the third day after injury the blood urea should be estimated and, in an unconscious patient, again two days later. If its level is raised, the feeding beyond the half-strength milk stage should be delayed until it has returned to normal. It is as well to check also the serum electrolytes (sodium, chloride and potassium) so that any abnormality may be corrected early but, provided adequate tube-feeding has not been too long delayed, it is only infrequently that there is much derangement. Restraint may be necessary at first to prevent the patient from pulling out his gastric tube, but its presence is usually soon tolerated. Sometimes fluid absorption by the gut is delayed for several days and it may be necessary to resort to intravenous infusion, although it should be remembered that a considerable amount of tap water can be absorbed from the rectum.

Gastric versus Intravenous Feeding

In the author's experience, the more natural route of feeding has, with the régime described below, proved altogether simpler and less troublesome than the intravenous, which requires closer control especially during the period of water- and sodium-retention.

Diabetes Insipidus

Injuries in the region of the tuber cinereum can result in diabetes insipidus, when very large quantities of urine may be passed (p. 63). The onset of this state is usually delayed until several days after the injury. Intake and output charts are therefore particularly important, since the depressed level of the patient's consciousness may not allow him to exhibit thirst.

Satisfy Thirst

Thirst in a stuporous patient who cannot ask for water is a cause of severe restlessness and must be satisfied. Urine from unconscious males may be collected through a length of Paul's rubber tubing strapped over the penis, or a condom with the end of its teat cut off and joined to a length of tubing. Only if there is bladder distension need a catheter be passed, for this is rarely necessary or desirable. In the female, however, an indwelling catheter, of the Foley type, may be used. These measures reduce much time-consuming changing of sheets, and prevent the skin of the hips, buttocks and sacrum being almost continuously soaked with urine.

Condom Urinary Drainage

Feeding.—All necessary nourishment can be provided through the gastric tube until the swallowing reflex has fully returned. When half-strength milk has been absorbed for thirty-six hours, and provided the blood urea is not much raised, full-strength milk is given. Twenty-four hours later (on approximately the fifth day after the injury) the katabolic phase is usually over and a fluid diet containing all essential foodstuffs, such as that provided by Complan, can be achieved in most cases. A summary of this feeding régime is given below in the form of a table. This, it is emphasized, is only a rough guide and should not be rigidly applied without regard to the individual patient's needs. Katabolism may be excessive and prolonged in some cases of severe brain injury, and however much protein is given, the body may fail to utilize it, and progressive wasting ensues. It is then worth trying one of the anabolic drugs, such as methandienone (Dianabol), though they are not usually effective. Loss of flesh and fat over the hips and sacrum will call for extra vigilance, since pressure sores are more likely to occur. Persistent lowering of the plasma proteins (which may show albumin/globulin reversal) and anaemia may require blood transfusion.

A Suggested Feeding Régime

<table>
<tr><th>Hours after Injury</th><th>Food</th><th>Quantity</th></tr>
<tr><td>0–20</td><td>Nil</td><td>Nil</td></tr>
<tr><td>20–24</td><td>Tap water</td><td>30 ml. hourly</td></tr>
<tr><td>24–36</td><td>,, ,,</td><td>60 ml. ,,</td></tr>
<tr><td>36–48</td><td>10% glucose-water</td><td>90 ml. ,,</td></tr>
<tr><td>48–84</td><td>50% milk in 10% glucose-water</td><td rowspan="3">90 ml. hourly increasing to 120 ml. hourly or 240 ml. 2-hourly.</td></tr>
<tr><td>84–108</td><td>Full-strength milk</td></tr>
<tr><td>108 (5th day) onwards</td><td>Complan</td></tr>
</table>

The Less Severely Injured

In the milder and fortunately much more usual case of head injury, physical recovery commonly proceeds uneventfully and a return to rational behaviour and complete orientation is fairly rapid. Sympathy is needed because it is a most bewildering experience to awaken slowly, as from a dream, in the strange environment of a hospital ward, particularly if one's last memory was, for example, one of returning speedily and joyfully from a dance in the front seat of a sports car. Repeated reassurance during this transition, and a simple explanation of what has happened, will make a great deal of difference to the patient and to her confidence in herself and in those who are looking after her. Some headache is of course common, and neck stiffness and Kernig's sign should be sought to see if there is meningism.

Lumbar Puncture

Lumbar Puncture

In my opinion, lumbar puncture has very little place in the management, the diagnosis or the treatment of head injuries. Moreover, in the early stages it has distinct dangers: a worsening of the patient's condition or even death may follow it if there happens to be an unrecognized intracranial clot, or if there is increased pressure due to brain swelling or contusion. It is a potentially dangerous method of detecting or relieving increased intracranial pressure, and it is not helpful in the early stages to know that the c.s.f. is bloodstained—an intracranial clot can exist with or without bloody c.s.f., and bloody c.s.f. is commonly present without a significant haematoma within the skull.

Two Indications

There are *two indications* for lumbar puncture. First, it should always be performed promptly at any time that bacterial meningitis is suspected, because the prognosis of this complication depends mostly on the speed with which treatment is instituted. Second, a less important indication, it may be carried out late in the first or in the second week after injury in patients who complain of persistent headache, *but who have no other suggestion of an intracranial haematoma*, such as drowsiness, bradycardia, papilloedema or vomiting, and in whom the clinical evidence of meningism has perhaps been equivocal. In this way, the presence of bloodstaining or, by then, a yellowish discoloration of the c.s.f., is detected, and the pace of the convalescence may be adjusted accordingly: those who have suffered subarachnoid haemorrhage require a more gradual rehabilitation; the others may with confidence be more firmly encouraged to increase their activities. Occasionally, the c.s.f. is found to be clear in patients with meningism, in which case convalescence can usually be accelerated.

Headache

It is surprising that headache should be so uncommonly a serious complaint in the early days immediately following a head injury, and yet may become a persistent one later (p. 79). *Severe headache in the early stages should always raise the suspicion of a complication.* Most headaches suffered after return to consciousness do not, however, commonly require for their relief anything stronger than aspirin or one of the many preparations containing this drug with phenacetin and codeine or caffeine. Full doses should be given and may even be judiciously exceeded when circumstances appear to warrant this. One meets sometimes a reluctance to prescribe and administer enough of this most useful drug at the very time when it is so useful, and this is strange when one reflects on the large doses taken by members of the general public when indulging in self-medication for lesser complaints.

Full Doses of Aspirin p.r.n.

Return to the upright posture after a head injury should be a graduated process. There is no doubt that this rule makes for smoother convalescence and fewer relapses than if patients are left to their own devices, bullied into early activity, or, as was once a fashion, kept flat in bed for one or two weeks in a room with drawn curtains.

Mobilization

Reactivation

There is considerable individual variation in the reaction to head injury and in the pace at which a patient can be restored to normal activity. The following scheme should be applied to even the mildest cases, because these may be just as difficult to rehabilitate as those that are more serious. Headache is the most reliable guide. As soon as it has ceased to be troublesome, a second pillow may be given, and the same evening or on the following day a back-rest, so that the patient can sit up in bed. If either of these stages is not tolerated owing to the return of headache or of other symptoms such as 'light-headedness' or definite vertigo, there should be reversion to the previous stage and a fresh start made more gradually the following day. It will usually be about two days after the cessation of headache before a patient is ready to sit out of bed for the first time—and twenty to thirty minutes is long enough for this occasion. Thereafter, increasing activity each day follows, whether in hospital or at home, so that the mildest case with less than an hour's P.T.A. will usually be in bed for about two days and back to full activity and work in about a week or two. It is equally important to initiate the process of resuming the upright posture as soon as the patient is ready, because being too long in bed may retard the patient's progress as much as getting up too soon.

Sitting up

Gradually Increased Activity

Consider what may happen if the programme for the patient is otherwise than that described; the case is typical of many on record. A man sustains 'mild concussion' during a football game, declines medical attention and returns to his home. He retires to bed early because of headache, and the following morning, although he does not feel really well, he is 'determined to shake it off', gets up and goes to work. He is forced to return home in the afternoon because he feels very much worse, and retires to bed. After several days in bed he feels very much better and gets straight up, only to suffer another set-back because of 'lightheadedness' and further headache. By now his confidence has become badly shaken, and understandably so. 'Loss of confidence' (there is no better term) is a potent source of invalidism and difficulty in returning to work, and the seeds of neurosis (p. 77) may be firmly sown at this stage, so that the patient takes perhaps two months to return to work instead of one or two weeks.

Careful *supervision* of the patient is of great importance. If each attempt to return to normal is met by a recurrence of symptoms, a patient must find it difficult to believe that he has not suffered serious damage. It is most important that we should not allow this to happen. He who has made a false start will do much better by cutting his losses and starting again entirely from scratch. One, then two pillows, a backrest, sitting up in a chair, and so on—*gradually*. This is most easily carried out in a hospital ward.

Why put them all to Bed?

In the case of the mildly injured patient, without serious symptoms, who is admitted purely for observation, there may be no good reason for requiring him to lie routinely in bed by day. The necessary observations can be carried out with the patient sitting in a chair.

Chapter 4

COMPLICATIONS

HERE, the direct complications of the injury will be considered, rather than those attending unconsciousness itself which were described in the previous chapter. For practical purposes, they may be divided into two groups: *Those requiring surgical treatment*, usually as a matter of some urgency; and *those whose treatment is not primarily surgical*, but which are serious, e.g., meningitis. At any time, a patient who is apparently progressing satisfactorily may relapse and succumb rapidly to either of these types of complication. To these a third group will be added, *Injuries to cranial nerves* which are, of course, part of the original injury, but it is convenient to consider them also in this chapter.

COMPLICATIONS DEMANDING SURGERY

1. Compound (Open) Depressed Skull Fractures

The primary objective of surgery here is to prevent infection reaching the intracranial cavity where, in spite of chemotherapy and antibiotics, greater havoc may be wrought than in almost any other part of the body. Prophylactic sulphadiazine should be started immediately (2 grammes stat.; 1 gramme four-hourly).

Chemotherapy and Antibiotics

This drug enters the c.s.f. in high concentration, but great care must be taken to maintain an adequate fluid intake and to keep the urine alkaline. Penicillin does not cross the 'blood-brain barrier' sufficiently, and it is questionable whether in the external tissues it is still a satisfactory antibiotic for prophylaxis, since hospital organisms now so often prove to be resistant to it. Many do not believe that this kind of prophylaxis is desirable, but in my view, the special danger of intracranial infection justifies the use of antibiotics, such as cloxacillin (Orbenin) with ampicillin (500 mg. of each, six-hourly) for this purpose, *but for a limited period of five days only in the first instance.*

There is no great urgency to operate on a compound depressed skull fracture which is uncomplicated by intracranial haemorrhage and cerebral compression, provided that the wound is covered and prophylactic drug therapy started promptly. If there are other aspects of the injury to be attended to, and particularly if the patient's general condition is unsatisfactory, the operation may be done at any time within the first twenty-four hours without a significantly increased risk of infection. If for any reason it is not possible to do a full operation within this period, it is usually better to carry out thorough excision of the scalp wound, which should then be closed against bacterial invaders. But the bone work and deeper exploration must be carried out later.

X-ray Assessment

Before operating on the fracture, its extent should be carefully assessed radiologically (p. 23), and it must be noted whether it is likely to be depressed into the lumen of the superior longitudinal or lateral venous sinuses, from which severe haemorrhage should be anticipated (see p. 51).

Local Analgesia

The operation is performed if possible under local analgesia, unless the patient has regained consciousness, or has never been unconscious, as may sometimes happen, particularly in the case of a frontal depressed fracture. The analgesia (p. 25) should extend beyond the confines of the scalp wound in any direction where an enlargement of, or a branch from, the incision may be necessary for the purpose of exposure. A generous removal of the hair should allow for this.

Test Scalp Mobility

The mobility of the scalp should be tested before the local anaesthetic is infiltrated, in order to see how much excision of the scalp edges can be afforded. If possible, the wound is better excised straight down to the bone. Curved haemostats are applied *to the aponeurosis* opposite bleeding points and allowed to hang over the scalp edges, or they are gathered and secured in a bunch, when their weight and leverage will obliterate the lumina of the blood vessels. One or two self-retaining retractors, of the toothed mastoidectomy type, are then inserted to help to control the haemorrhage and to allow a full exposure of the depression and its margins. All visible dirt, hair, etc., must be removed, together with contaminated pericranium. A burr-hole is made through unfractured bone adjacent to the fracture, and enlarged if necessary to allow the depressed fragments to be elevated. The two tables of the skull will usually have been split into unequal flakes and the inner ones pushed under the edge of the intact bone. Loose fragments should be removed cautiously and gently, and not rocked or rotated, lest the dura and brain beneath be further damaged. All loose and contaminated pieces should be removed; those still attached to pericranium may be replaced if not dirty. Unclean edges of the intact skull should be nibbled away, and further bone removal may be necessary to expose fully a tear of the dura mater beneath, which, if contaminated, should also be trimmed. Any bone fragments or foreign material are then removed gently from the brain itself, after enlargement of the dural opening if this has been necessary. Bleeding cortical vessels are gently held in fine dissecting forceps which are touched by the electrode connected to the lightest diathermy current that will produce coagulation.

Gentle Technique

If the dural edges can be easily approximated, the tear is closed with fine silk sutures, but it is unnecessary to make a fetish, as some do, of closing a dural defect at all costs, provided that the superficial excision has been thorough and the scalp is closed properly. Bleeding points on the dura are lightly coagulated with the diathermy, and the scalp is sutured in two layers with black silk. An efficient dressing is then applied to keep out organisms, particularly those from the patient's fingers.

Hernia cerebri

Hernia cerebri, or brain fungus, results from infection of a penetrating wound and is facilitated by inefficient scalp closure. Similar in some ways to a burst abdomen, it is a dangerous condition for which specialist help should be sought.

2. Intracranial Haemorrhage

The importance of subarachnoid haemorrhage has already been stressed, but this does not call for operative treatment.

Extradural Haemorrhage

(a) Extradural (Middle Meningeal) Haemorrhage.— The circumstances and signs of this most grave and urgent complication have been told in Chapter 2 (pp. 10–15) and are given in surgical textbooks. They will not be repeated here, but three somewhat neglected features of the early stage, when the clot is developing, should be noted. One is *restlessness* which is common but by no means pathognomonic, and if the patient is conscious he usually complains bitterly of headache. The second is the rapid development of marked, boggy *oedema of the scalp*, localized over the site of the clot and overlying fracture; this is a very common feature, although again not decisive in favour of this diagnosis, as it may occur to some extent over the site of any fracture. Third is *a shift of the midline structures* of the brain, indicated in the plain x-rays by a calcified pineal or by the Echo-E.G. (p. 24).

The Operation

The operation must be done at the hospital where the condition is diagnosed and *as soon as it is diagnosed.* A brace and set of skull perforators and burrs, somebone rongeurs, diathermy and electric suction apparatus should be available (which they are not at present) in every hospital that admits head injuries. *The life-saving measure is to open the skull sufficiently to allow the clot to be extruded.*

Urgency

No time should be lost; many so-called emergencies are but relative—this one is absolute. The hair should be clipped as quickly as possible over the side of the dilating pupil, and this will usually reveal more clearly the boggy oedema forming over the fracture. An endotracheal tube should be passed. While the scalp is being shaved, the theatre and instruments are made ready and blood is urgently ordered, together with someone to administer it.

A burr-hole is made in the skull beneath the oedema, *close to the fracture*, and is enlarged sufficiently to gain a good exposure. *Nothing should prevent this from being done as soon as the scalp is prepared for the incision*—one should not wait for full sterilization of the instruments. In children, especially, there may be no fracture, and it may be necessary to make both anterior and posterior temporal burr-holes to expose first the anterior and then the posterior branches of the middle meningeal artery. The anterior one is best made low in the temporal fossa (see Fig. 7), in case the clot is largely beneath the temporal lobe and so that the main trunk of the middle meningeal artery can be reached. A good light is essential, and a pair of small self-retaining retractors will control a good deal of the bleeding from the superficial and deep temporal arteries and will save some time being wasted while these are attended to.

Usually there is a chief arterial bleeding point, but this will not be seen precisely until the clot has been scraped or sucked right off the dura mater. It is then most easily secured by means of the coagulating diathermy current, but if none is available a Cushing silver clip may be applied or the artery ligated by means of a transfixion suture through the dura mater. Only rarely is it necessary to try to follow the textbook advice to plug the foramen spinosum with a boiled matchstick; this is usually a very difficult procedure for anyone not familiar with this sort of operation and in the face of severe haemorrhage. If bleeding comes from the bone, it may be stopped with Horsley's wax.

Even after the main bleeding point has been secured, a great deal of haemorrhage may persist, but *most of this is congestive and secondary to the increased intracranial pressure which has now been eased, and it will gradually diminish spontaneously*, although it may be as much as an hour or more before it settles sufficiently to allow the wound to be closed. Provided lost blood is being replaced, one can afford to be patient.

I have now stopped trying to drain these wounds, believing this to be useless against clot which is usually insufficiently fluid to find its way outwards. It is a simple matter to reopen the wound the following day, or earlier if necessary, to evacuate a reaccumulation of haematoma, but it is unusual to have to do this. The signs of recurrence will be much the same as those that preceded the first operation, but, owing to the bony decompression, they will develop more slowly and allow more time for action.

Recurrent Bleeding

The temporal muscle and its fascial sheath should be sutured separately with silk, and the scalp also in two layers in the fashion already recommended. This careful closure will diminish the subsequent evidence of the bony defect and may save the necessity for cranioplasty later. Many neurosurgeons nowadays turn a bone flap for this condition, but this is not advised under the circumstances described, because it will take so much longer than the simpler, local craniectomy.

Having dealt with the important features of the operation that is needed, one must now recognize quite frankly that the conditions under which it has to be performed may well be far from ideal and that the task is one which few other than neurosurgeons care to undertake, however stern have been the enjoinders and precise the instructions in the textbooks and other writings. It is hoped that the suggestions here may encourage those who find themselves suddenly in what is an extremely responsible position.

Special Circumstances

You may be faced with a case of extradural haemorrhage under three main circumstances, which depend on who you are, where you are, and whether there is a neurosurgeon available to help you.

(i) *When you have inadequate facilities, with no option but to deal with it by yourself in the best way you can in order to save the patient's life.* You may even have no surgical instrument for opening the skull, although an old trephine can usually be found in most hospitals which have a theatre. If not, a carpenter's brace and bit can be used. Once the hole is made, there will be less difficulty in finding a tool (even a pair of pliers) with which to enlarge it. *The important thing is to open the skull* somehow, and quickly. If the inexperienced operator does no more than this, he may have done enough to save the patient's life, because a blood transfusion can be set up (another person should attend to this matter as soon as possible) and loss of blood counteracted. In this way a vital respite is gained, even if the operator finds it difficult to control the subsequent bleeding; for, with lost blood being replaced, he can pack the wound cavity until a neurosurgeon comes, or he can even transfer the patient in this safer condition to a neurosurgical unit, so that the operation can be completed. This has been done successfully.

Pack the Wound if necessary

(ii) *When you and your facilities are adequate to deal with the situation.* The operation should proceed as described.

Neurosurgical Aid

(iii) *When neurosurgical aid is available and desired,* there should be no hesitation in asking for it, provided the opening of the skull is not delayed. Such help can now generally be obtained by telephone throughout most of Britain, although distances may dictate that it consists only of advice. If the neurosurgeon is presented quickly and concisely with the relevant facts of the case, he will be able to decide what course of action offers the patient the best chance.

Speed in Diagnosis and Treatment

The mortality from extradural haemorrhage itself, apart from that due to associated brain damage, is directly dependent upon the speed with which the condition is recognized and how promptly the clot is evacuated. Somehow, surgical teaching has made too little impression on the lamentable death-rate from this often remediable condition—a mortality sometimes cruelly regarded as inevitable.

Ideally, the operation should be done by a neurosurgeon, but someone must first make the diagnosis, and *it will usually be for the surgeon on the spot to get started while the neurosurgeon comes to his aid as quickly as possible.*

(b) Subdural Haemorrhage.—This may be acute, subacute or chronic.

Acute Subdural Haemorrhage occurs rapidly after the injury; the 'lucid interval' may be only relative or not seen at all, because there is often severe brain damage as well. The patient who may have been responding to painful or lesser stimuli on admission soon ceases to do so, and exploratory burr-holes should be made (at least two on each side, if necessary) after the hair has been fully clipped. If the source of the haemorrhage is a large tear in a venous sinus, it may be difficult or impossible to locate and repair this in the face of haemorrhage that is usually much more severe than anything encountered extradurally. Elevation of the head will reduce the venous pressure and allow the tear to be sutured with less difficulty, or to be covered with Gelfoam or a muscle patch. This type of haemorrhage has an extremely high mortality; fortunately, it is not common.

A less severe form comes from superficial cerebral veins in a cerebral laceration, and may be remedied. An efficient suction apparatus is essential, and the hole in the skull must be adequate to admit a good light. Again, enlargement of the burr-hole with bone rongeurs is the most expeditious method of approach.

Subacute Subdural Haemorrhage occurs more insidiously during the early days following the injury, and this group merges with the more familiar *Chronic Subdural Haematoma*, which accumulates much more gradually, sometimes over a period of months. It is more likely to occur in elderly patients whose more shrunken brains allow the space for it and in whom the injury may have been trivial and often forgotten.

Headache is the predominant symptom. Localizing signs are indefinite and pupillary changes often absent, but there is usually a *deficiency or loss of conjugate upward movement of the eyes*, either in response to a command to look up, or, in stuporous patients, when the cornea is lightly touched while the lids are held open. There is often *bradycardia*, and a characteristic fluctuating, but eventually deteriorating level of responsiveness.

Burr-holes

Burr-holes.—The haematoma, particularly if chronic, is frequently bilateral, so that burr-holes should always be made on both sides. Usually frontal and parietal ones will locate the fluid, but temporal ones should also be made if none is found at the other sites (Fig. 7). Generally speaking, haematomas are more likely to be found in the acute stage through temporal burr-holes, and through frontal or parietal ones after the first two weeks.

Subdural Hygroma

Sometimes there is not a haematoma, but a *hygroma*, consisting usually of straw-coloured fluid

FIG. 7. (*see opposite.*)—Three suggested sites for burr-holes. The temporal hole should be *low* to avoid the lateral sulcus and the speech areas on the left side; it is usually made too high. Frontal and posterior parietal holes are in front of the coronal and lambdoid sutures on a parasagittal line which passes through the centre of the eye. If the position of the coronal suture cannot be seen or felt, it will be found 14 cm. from the nasion.

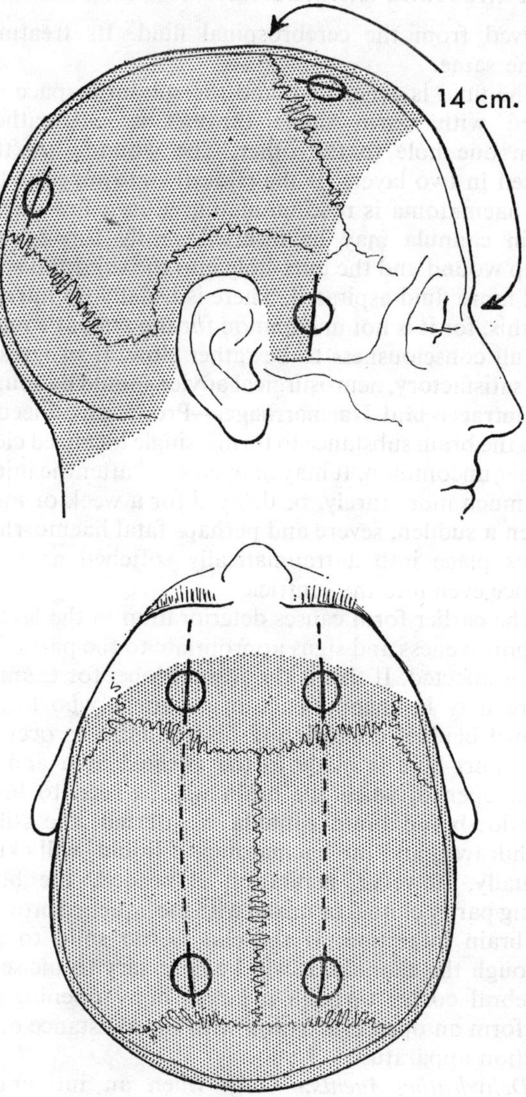

FIG. 7.

derived from the cerebrospinal fluid. Its treatment is the same.

The fluid is evacuated, and the subdural space irrigated with warm saline through a soft catheter from one hole to the other. The wounds are then closed in two layers. If the clinical state suggests that the haematoma is reaccumulating after a few days, a brain cannula may be inserted gently through the scalp wound and the burr-hole into the subdural space and more fluid aspirated. There is usually no hurry to do this, for it is not uncommon for the patient's return to full consciousness to be rather slow. If progress is not satisfactory, neurosurgical advice should be sought.

(c) Intracerebral Haemorrhage.—Progressive bleeding into the brain substance to form a single localized clot is rather uncommon. It may happen soon after the injury, or, much more rarely, be delayed for a week or more, when a sudden, severe and perhaps fatal haemorrhage takes place into a traumatically softened area and thence even into the ventricle.

The earlier form causes deterioration in the level of responsiveness and signs appropriate to the part of the brain affected. If this is the frontal lobe, for example, there may be incontinence in a patient who has regained bladder control, and fits are liable to occur.

A burr-hole is made in the affected area and the dura opened, when the brain will be seen to bulge. A wide-bored brain cannula is inserted, the stilette withdrawn, and the haematoma, if liquid, will exude. Usually, however, aspiration is needed, the blood being partly clotted or mixed with the liquefied products of brain infarction. If the clot is too solid to pass through the cannula, it will be necessary to incise the cerebral cortex through a larger bony opening and perform an open evacuation with the assistance of the suction apparatus.

Dehydrating Agents.—Only when an intracranial haematoma has been excluded should consideration be given to the reduction of increased intracranial pressure due to brain swelling (cerebral 'oedema') by means of strong dehydrating agents. Such swelling results from respiratory obstruction, prolonged arterial hypotension and other conditions which lead to anoxia and increased capillary permeability, and it accompanies contusion, haemorrhage and infarction. These conditions should therefore be prevented or remedied whereever possible, for they are not removed simply by treating their effect. Provided this is understood, there is sometimes a place for large doses of dexamethasone *Steroids* (Decadron), given intravenously, 10 mg. stat.; 4 mg. six-hourly for 48 hours; thereafter reducing the dosage and discontinuing after 5 days. For a more rapid effect, intravenous urea (Urevert) or mannitol may be tried.

The main indication for dehydrating measures is when the patient's level of responsiveness is deteriorating and burr-holes have revealed a tight bulging brain, but no haematoma.

3. Intracranial Abscess

This complication, which may be extradural, subdural or intracerebral, is now fortunately rare, because it can nearly always be prevented. Its detection may be difficult, but it should be suspected if meningitis (p. 61–63) fails to resolve fully, the increased white cells in the c.s.f. being accompanied by a rising protein content. Cases where there has been inadequate or late wound débridement, and particularly those with infected scalp wounds, should be watched closely for the development of signs and symptoms of increased intracranial pressure. The infection may either pass directly from scalp or air sinuses to brain via a septic thrombosis in an emissary vein, or localize more superficially within the cranium. An intracranial haematoma may become infected via the bloodstream; in

Percivall Pott's day, extradural infection in the presence of an intact scalp seems to have been not an infrequent complication of head trauma, but now such a thing, with a 'puffy tumour', is rare, perhaps owing to the relative infrequency elsewhere in the body of pre-existing external and other septic foci causing bacteraemia. If an abscess is suspected, the patient should be transferred to a neurosurgical unit, for this condition requires specialized management.

4. Skull Defects

These should not normally be repaired until the wound has been soundly healed for several months, and this operation is also better undertaken in a neurosurgical unit. Plastic substances are now available and are easier to fashion than a tantalum plate, and may sometimes be inserted into a clean wound at the primary operation.

Special Aids to Diagnosis

Intentionally, there has been no mention of the electro-encephalogram, of carotid angiography, isotope brain scans, air encephalography, or ventriculography. These investigations are properly adjuncts to specialized neurosurgical practice with which this book is not concerned; their results can mislead even the initiated, and much valuable time can be lost if they are attempted in hospitals which are not geared to their routine use. The use and limitations of the Echo-E.G. have been mentioned on p. 24. Later on, when a patient is not recovering as well as it is felt he should be, special aid may seem a desirable alternative, in the absence of localizing signs, to resorting to the 'woodpecker' method of multiple burr-holes. Under these circumstances, it is again better to transfer the case, for there is usually plenty of time to arrange this.

Making Burr-Holes

It will be as well at this stage to summarize some points about the siting of burr-holes:

(1) It is usually best to make the first hole adjacent to any fracture and, if it is a long fracture, a hole at each end of it.
(2) If one pupil has become dilated, any haematoma will usually be on the same side.
(3) In the first hours or days, any haematoma will usually be on the side opposite a hemiplegia. Later, a chronic subdural haematoma may be on either side or on both sides.
(4) In these early stages, haematomas are more often found towards the base of the skull than nearer the vertex. Hence the importance of the *low* temporal burr-hole.
(5) It is easier to learn *how* to make a burr-hole than to know *when* and *where* to make it.
(6) As with any technical procedure, reading about it is no substitute for seeing it performed. Practice on cadavers is recommended.

Serious Complications not demanding Urgent Surgery

1. Epileptic Fits may occur at any stage after a head injury, and some head injuries are of course the result of an epileptic person's falling, although this may not have been realized initially. Fits are most disquieting events to those not used to dealing with them, and they are not always recognized for what they are. It is not possible here to discuss their almost infinite variety. The essential feature is a *sudden* deterioration, usually of consciousness, and usually, but not always, with convulsive movements. It is when the initial stages pass unobserved that it may not be realized what has happened. Normally, some recovery in the level of responsiveness follows shortly, but it should be emphasized that, if the brain is already contused or lacerated, the period of anoxia and venous congestion that attends an apnoeic phase in a fit may result in a more lasting deterioration. Moreover, if a fit is heralding clot-compression of the brain, the progressive deterioration that would in any case follow may be much accelerated, and remedial action must also be more rapid. Usually, however, fits are merely a response of certain brains to the injury and do not *by themselves* necessarily indicate a particular complication.

The Significance of Fits

Since fits may be the source of further damage to an injured brain, they should be treated *promptly*, with the object of preventing further attacks and, particularly, *status epilepticus, which may be lethal.* When they occur, further anxiety arises from having to break the rule which normally should prevent us from lowering the patient's level of responsiveness artificially with drugs. But this now has to be done, and an even greater vigilance will be required to detect intracranial bleeding.

If the fits are minor ones, such as the slight twitchings of the face that sometimes occur and which are not accompanied by a detectable deterioration in the level of responsiveness or by respiratory embarrassment, it is unnecessary to take drastic action. Phenytoin sodium (Epanutin) 100 mg. should be given intramuscularly and then 50 mg. six-hourly by mouth or tube; this drug is almost purely anticonvulsant in its action and causes very little depression of consciousness. However, the barbiturate, sodium amytal, 30–180 mg. intramuscularly, is usually a better drug for controlling fits in children.

Phenytoin Sodium

If there are more disturbing convulsions, these must be stopped promptly lest the dangerous complication of status epilepticus should develop. Phenytoin sodium (Epanutin) 100 mg. should be given intravenously in addition to the intramuscular dose al-

Status Epilepticus

ready mentioned. If this proves ineffective, diazepam (Valium) 5 mg. intravenously and 5 mg. intramuscularly should be added. If frequent fits still continue, it is probably best then to resort to endoctracheal intubation, curarization and controlled respiration. This will ensure that the airway remains clear in the face of any convulsions that may break through the paralysing agents, and is safer than the former practice of giving large doses of paraldehyde by intravenous drip (50 ml. in 568 ml. of 5 per cent glucose solution).

Phenobarbitone, even when given intramuscularly, is not usually sufficiently rapid in its action to deal with this sort of situation, and its use is not recommended. Moreover the cumulative effect of repeated doses is liable to be a profound lowering of the level of responsiveness later.

Late traumatic epilepsy is considered on p. 81.

2. C.S.F. Rhinorrhoea and Otorrhoea.—The former is much the less uncommon; it rarely persists for more than a few days and no active measures are advisable to try to stop it. It must be distinguished from the serous secretion of the nasal mucosa which is sometimes excessive, particularly in those subject to allergic rhinitis, but which only rarely soaks the pillow and handkerchiefs in the way that c.s.f. does. When there is doubt, the fluid may be collected and tested *fresh* for sugar, which is not present in significant quantity in nasal secretion, and for mucin, which is. But more striking confirmation is provided by the greatly increased flow of c.s.f. which may occur if the head is lowered in the prone position and the jugular veins compressed.

No Nose-blowing

The patient, if conscious, is forbidden to sit up or to blow his nose. This is to prevent a reversal of the flow in the fistula from the potentially infected nasal cavities to the subarachnoid space. It should be realized that the intracranial c.s.f. pressure in these cases is, in a recumbent patient, almost zero, and that if lumbar puncture should be performed the withdrawal of fluid may also cause this reversal of flow. I have twice seen meningitis follow within a few hours of such injudicious interference. This does not mean that lumbar puncture, for the purpose of diagnosis and treatment, should be withheld if there is a reasonable suspicion that meningitis has in fact occurred; some calculated risks must be taken.

A rare consequence of a c.s.f. leak is that an intracranial clot may develop unusually insidiously owing to the decompressive effect of the fistula.

Barrier-nursing should be instituted when there is c.s.f. leakage, attendants and visitors wearing masks. Prophylactic sulphadiazine, 2 grammes stat.; 1 gramme four-hourly, should be given by mouth (or by gastric tube), and meningitis constantly anticipated. The patient should receive a substantial fluid intake, and enough potassium citrate to render the urine alkaline. The urine should be tested daily for acidity and for blood, because sulphadiazine will crystallize in acid urine, causing haematuria and even anuria. Antibiotics are unnecessary unless c.s.f. is coming through an infected nose or ear. Plugs should not be put in the nose or ears; it is better to allow the infected external pathway to be washed out with the weak sulphonamide solution of the c.s.f. If the flow appears unduly profuse and persistent, the head should be elevated in order to reduce it but, for the reasons already mentioned, a slightly positive pressure within the cranium should always be encouraged.

Two days after the c.s.f. leakage appears to have ceased, and cannot be restarted by the jugular-compression test, all prophylactic treatment is discontinued. If, however, the rhinorrhoea or otorrhoea persist for more than a week, neurosurgical advice should be obtained.

Traumatic Pneumocephalus.—Air may enter the cranial cavity if c.s.f. is escaping, but sometimes this occurs without associated rhinorrhoea. It is an uncommon occurrence, but will be detected if the skull is x-rayed routinely, when the films reveal air in the subdural or subarachnoid space, in the ventricles, or an aërocele in the brain itself. Sometimes the amount of air is so small that it is either overlooked or does not allow certain identification, and it is as well, in cases of doubt, to repeat the examination in a few days. Usually subdural and subarachnoid air will have absorbed by then, but very occasionally the rare condition of a tension pneumocephalus develops and will require the release of air under pressure by means of a cannula inserted through a burr-hole.

When they have sufficiently recovered, patients should have any large dural fistula repaired with a graft of fascia lata, since the risk of meningitis later is a serious one. They should be referred to a neurosurgical unit for this operation.

Where c.s.f. rhinorrhoea is associated with a central maxillary fracture, it may happen that the c.s.f. flow ceases at about the same time that the fracture is reduced. There is no evidence that this is other than coincidence. Most c.s.f. leaks stop spontaneously within a few days, and it is hard to see how reducing the fracture could close a meningeal tear; the manipulation would be as likely to extend it.

3. Meningitis must be recognized and treated promptly, the prognosis depending on the speed of diagnosis and treatment. Headache is usually severe and there is restlessness, photophobia, often vomiting and sometimes seizures. High fever, neck stiffness and Kernig's sign are found on examination. The diagnosis is confirmed immediately by discovering turbid c.s.f. at lumbar puncture, when intrathecal treatment should be started at the same time, without waiting for the pathological examination of the fluid.

Intrathecal Antibiotics

When its origin is from the nose, post-traumatic

meningitis is usually due to the pneumococcus, which is nearly always sensitive to penicillin. This antibiotic should be given intramuscularly (2 mega-units stat.; 1 mega-unit six-hourly) to deal with the organisms in the air sinuses, and by lumbar puncture (20,000 units initially and then 10,000 units daily for at least 7 days in a concentration of 2,000 units per 1 ml. of doubly-distilled, pyrogen-free water or normal saline) to allow immediate and direct access to the infected c.s.f. *This dosage is most important:* the Sunday newspapers at one time used to bear witness to the fatal outcome that may attend the administration of ten times or more the proper intrathecal dosage. If there is also c.s.f. rhinorrhoea, it will usually be advisable to give penicillin intrathecally *twice* daily because of the loss of the drug in the leaking fluid.

If the organism is insensitive to penicillin, streptomycin should be given, 1 gramme systemically per day and 50 mg. in 1 ml. intrathecally. There are few organisms that do not respond to the combination of these two drugs given intrathecally, by which route a high concentration is achieved compared with that obtained via the choroid plexuses by intramuscular dosage alone.

It is advisable also to give sulphadiazine (3 grammes stat.; 1·5 grammes four-hourly) in addition to antibiotics; *but plenty of fluid must be given and the urine kept alkaline* (with potassium citrate) to avoid crystal deposits. The drug is administered orally or by tube, unless the patient is vomiting when Sulphamezathine (sulphadimidine) should be given intravenously or intramuscularly in the same dosage.

An alternative to intrathecal antibiotic treatment is to give Sulphamezathine (sulphadimidine) or very high doses of penicillin continuously by intravenous drip. The author however prefers, in the intrathecal (or intraventricular) route, the certainty of an immediate exposure of the organisms to a very high concentration of antibiotic to a slower and less certain concentration achieved indirectly through the choroid plexuses. Speed of action, both by doctor and by drugs, appears to be the most important factor in the combating of meningitis and its complications.

Epanutin (50 mg. eight-hourly) should be given as prophylaxis against fits.

4. Hyperpyrexia must be emphasized again here; its management has already been fully described on pp. 35–36.

5. Metabolic Disorders.—It is advisable to check the blood urea and electrolytes on the third and fifth days after injury so that adjustments in the feeding arrangements can be made in good time before any imbalance gets out of hand (pp. 36–39). It should be remembered that the blood urea may show a moderate rise in the presence of a chest infection or a large haematoma.

6. Diabetes Insipidus has also been mentioned (p. 38). It is important to recognize the excessive urinary output and to see that fluid intake is adequate. If it persists for more than a few days, substitution therapy with antidiuretic hormone should be given in the form of injections of Pitressin tannate in oil; the dosage must be determined by trial: usually 1 ml. (5 pressor units) daily or every two days is sufficient to bring the water exchange within reasonable limits. If the disability is prolonged or permanent, special snuff containing dried posterior pituitary extract (Di-Sipidin) or a Lysine-vasopressin nasal spray (Sandoz) may be tried as alternatives to injection therapy.

7. Skull Fractures.—The fractures that are of special significance by virtue of the complications they may produce have been mentioned already: compound depressed fractures; linear ones that cross the middle meningeal artery and its branches; and those involving the air sinuses. These have not in themselves been emphasized because, from the practical point of view, their importance is small compared with the complications that may result from them: intracranial infection, extradural haemorrhage, and c.s.f. leakage, meningitis and aërocele.

Other fractures are of even less importance *per se*. Simple localized depressed fractures, especially in children, may be elevated without urgency by making a small burr-hole close to the depression and introducing a suitable elevator between the skull and dura mater. In infants, a burr-hole may be unnecessary if the pericranium and dura can be carefully separated from the margins of the open anterior fontanelle by sharp dissection in order to allow the elevator access to a depression (a 'pond' fracture) in the vicinity. This is really a cosmetic and psychological matter, for there is little convincing evidence that the continuing presence of a simple depression in the skull is otherwise harmful; when trouble, notably epilepsy, develops, it is a result of damage done at the time of injury, which is not undone by elevating the fracture. For the rest of the fractures, we may join Pott in dismissing the practice of dividing them into different sorts: "These are to be found in most of the old books, but as they merely load the memory, without informing the understanding, or assisting the practitioner, modern authors have generally laid them aside."

8. Traumatic Cephalhydrocele or 'Meningocele'.—Occasionally c.s.f. will find its way out through a tear in the meninges and a linear fracture into the subpericranial or subaponeurotic layer beneath an intact scalp. This seems to occur particularly in young children, and the fluctuant swelling it produces may be differentiated from a haematoma if transillumination can be demonstrated and an impulse on coughing. If it does not subside spontaneously after a few days, it is safer to reduce it by means of lumbar puncture than by direct aspiration. Afterwards a pad is placed over its site and secured by a firm crêpe bandage.

9. Carotid-cavernous Fistula.—This rare but intriguing

complication may follow injury to the internal carotid artery within the cavernous sinus. Usually there is a delay of a few days or even weeks before the weakened wall gives way and an arteriovenous fistula is established. The patient may notice the resulting bruit, or be quite unaware of it, even though it can be heard clearly through a stethoscope applied to the closed eye or the supra-orbital region. Unilateral pulsating exophthalmos then occurs, or it may be bilateral if the fistula is a large one and if the intercavernous sinuses are well developed. Chemosis and ophthalmoplegia may also follow, and, if the arterialization of the blood in the conjunctival venules is not recognized as such, the red eye may be mistaken for that of conjunctivitis. There is no hurry to attempt surgical treatment, for this is not always satisfactory and some of these fistulae appear to be unstable and will close spontaneously, or when provoked to do so by an episode of arterial hypotension or by the irritation of carotid angiography. The treatment of this complication is a controversial subject, and a specialist opinion should be sought.

Two unusual conditions may be met which, although not complications of the injury to the head, may be mistaken for them.

Cerebral Fat Embolism.—This occurs usually about twelve to seventy-two hours after injury. Typically, there is a major limb or pelvic fracture. Initial lung embolization gives rise to tachypnoea, tachycardia and fever, which may be ascribed to 'inhalation pneumonia'. A patient who has regained, or who has never lost, consciousness becomes confused and restless, even delirious, and in severe cases stupor, coma and death may follow. The initial confused wakefulness and tachycardia are unusual features of cerebral compression, and lumbar puncture will exclude meningitis, which may also be suspected. The characteristic petechiae around the shoulders and thorax should be sought.

There is no specific treatment, nor any of certain efficacy; but energetic attention to the associated respiratory insufficiency is clearly important.

Traumatic Internal Carotid Thrombosis.—The combination of an injury to the chin and angle of the mandible with a fractured sternum may stretch and tear the internal carotid artery in the neck. Thrombosis, followed by embolism to the middle cerebral artery may then result in cerebral infarction and hemiplegia some hours after injury. Initially, there is no evidence of increased intracranial pressure, but the prognosis is uncertain and death may follow from uncontrollable brain swelling.

Injuries to Cranial Nerves

These injuries, which do not require urgent surgical attention, may conveniently be considered here, although they are part of the initial injury rather than true complications. They will usually have been noted at the examination in the casualty department, but may be better assessed later in the ward, after more pressing matters have been attended to.

I. Anosmia.—When the nostrils have become free from obstruction and the patient is no longer confused, the function of the first cranial nerve should be tested with odours such as oil of cloves, peppermint, camphor, and tincture of asafoetida. This cranial nerve is the one most commonly injured, and some degree of hyposmia, on one or both sides, is not infrequent. Complete loss of the sense of smell, with which there may be some apparent interference with taste, is usually permanent and nothing can be done to influence its recovery. Some regard this as but a minor inconvenience, while to others it is a serious misfortune. The late Mr. Justice Lynskey, in awarding damages to an unfortunate sufferer from this disability, recognized that it was "a loss of one of the delights of life". In an appendix to this book, Brian Elliott gives a vivid and moving account of what this means to him. An important domestic consequence of anosmia used to be the inability to detect coal gas.

II. The Optic Nerve may be contused or even transected at the optic foramen in association with an adjacent fracture which may be difficult to demonstrate radiologically, even with special views. Vision may be completely lost; or partially, with scotomata demonstrable in the visual field of the affected eye. The direct pupillary light reflex will be correspondingly lost or depressed, while the consensual reaction is preserved on the affected side; these reactions of the pupils distinguish a second- from a third-cranial nerve injury when the patient is unconscious (Figs. 2–5). The question of 'decompression' of the optic nerve in its canal is sometimes raised, but there is probably no significant compression. The operation is technically difficult, and may well result in added damage. The position is much the same as with closed depressed fractures affecting the brain and spinal cord—the damage is nearly always done at the time of the injury by contusion or laceration, and operation is no remedy. Sometimes quite useful recovery of vision occurs, particularly in partial lesions, but this cannot be predicted.

Chiasmal Damage

Sometimes the chiasma is damaged, in which case bitemporal hemianopia will result. As might be expected, such a lesion may be associated with diabetes insipidus from damage to the neighbouring region of the tuber cinereum (p. 63).

III, IV and VI. The Oculomotor, Trochlear and Abducent Nerves may be damaged singly, or in combination within the orbit or cavernous sinus. Occasionally, the abducens shows loss of function some time after the initial injury, as it may also do, rarely, after lumbar puncture or a spontaneous subarachnoid haemorrhage; the precise mechanism of this delayed process is not clear (see also p. 17).

Several months should be allowed for recovery of external ophthalmoplegia before operations on the external ocular muscles are attempted to correct diplopia or the appearance of a squint. Many cases make a good spontaneous recovery. One of Nature's inefficiencies is that the function of the levator palpebrae usually recovers before that of those external ocular muscles which are also supplied by the third

Diplopia

nerve, and this may result in troublesome diplopia as soon as the ptosis improves sufficiently to allow vision

Eye-patch

in that eye. If diplopia is annoying, a patch should be worn, and this may be alternated between the normal and the affected eye until binocular vision is restored. Not all people have true binocular vision, and others are able to suppress the false image, in which cases a severe squint may cause no inconvenience.

In cases of orbital injury, it is often the extrinsic muscles themselves that are damaged, rather than their nerves.

V. The Trigeminal Nerve or, more precisely, one of its branches is occasionally injured. The infra-orbital nerve is particularly affected, usually in association with a fracture of the zygomatic bone or maxilla which may be hidden by facial swelling, but revealed by the presence of anaesthesia of the upper lip. The supraorbital nerve is not infrequently contused in direct frontal soft-tissue injuries. A fracture of the middle cranial fossa may damage parts of the trigeminal complex more proximally, or the gasserian ganglion itself. Recovery may be incomplete and the altered sensation a source of annoyance and sometimes obsession.

VII. Facial Paralysis, due to injury of the lower motor neurones of the seventh cranial nerve, may be *immediate* or its appearance may be *delayed* for several days. In the first instance there is often anatomical disruption of the nerve within its bony canal which is fractured, in which case there may be only incomplete regeneration, or none at all. At least a year should be allowed for recovery before corrective measures, such as nerve anastomosis or plastic sling operations, are attempted. External facial splints are useful in theory, but are usually so uncomfortable that patients, once away from hospital, discard them and their added unsightliness with relief. If something is felt to be necessary to boost the patient's morale, intermittent galvanic stimulation of the affected muscles is dramatic treatment and will do no harm, but it has now been shown that this in no way influences the degree or rapidity of recovery.

The *delayed form of paralysis* appears usually within a week of the injury, sometimes, to the consternation of the patient, after he has been sent home. It is possible that there is delayed oedema of the nerve within its sheath, resulting in ischaemia, or compression by subsequent bleeding in the canal or by fluid attracted by osmosis to the breakdown products of the blood. Unlike the immediate type of paralysis, the prognosis here is good and recovery the rule, for the nerve is anatomically intact. This accounts for the success of some operations that have been undertaken to decompress the nerve, but attempts to do this by anyone who is not skilled at this delicate procedure are to be severely discouraged, because the effect may be the opposite to that intended.

If the face is much injured and swollen, or if the patient is deeply unconscious, an immediate facial palsy may not be recognized, and when seen later may be mistaken for a delayed one. From the point of view of prognosis, therefore, facial paralysis should be sought early by observing the response of the face to the pain of bilateral supra-orbital pressure.

When the nerve branch to the stapedius muscle is affected by the injury, there may occasionally be troublesome hyperacusis but this usually clears up after a few days. Those who wish to exercise further their knowledge of the anatomy of the facial nerve may look for disturbance of tear secretion and also discover whether the injury is proximal or distal to the point where the chorda tympani leaves it, by testing the sense of taste on the anterior two-thirds of the tongue.

VIII. The Auditory Nerve itself is probably not often damaged; disturbance of hearing after a head injury is usually a defect of conduction. The cochlea itself, however, may be involved in a petrous bone fracture.

Similarly, the vestibular end-organ is damaged rather than its nerve and this may result in definite vertigo

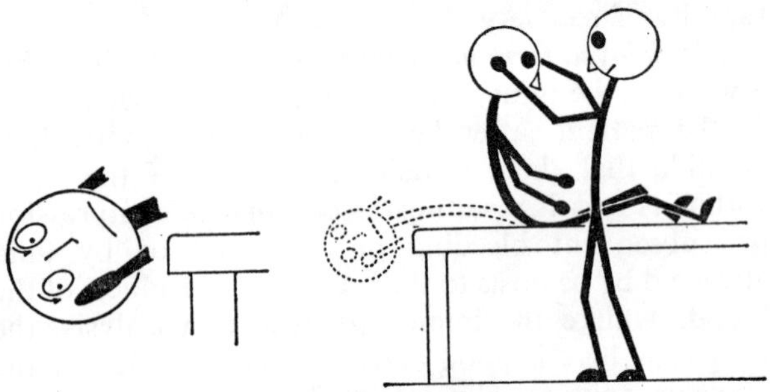

FIG. 8.—A test for positional vertigo.

when the head is moved into certain positions, particularly backwards and to one side. The test for such damage is illustrated in Fig. 8. The patient is seated on a couch and the examiner turns the head some 30°–45° to one side and then lowers it briskly to about 30° below the horizontal. After a brief latent period, there is vertigo and distress, with rotatory and horizontal nystagmus towards the undermost ear if the utricle on that side has been damaged. If there is no response, the manoeuvre is repeated after a short interval, with the head turned to the opposite side.

The importance of this test is that it may provide the only physical sign that there is an organic cause for the vertigo, and indicate that the symptom is not a 'neurotic' one (p. 78). Treatment consists of reassurance and telling the patient to avoid this position of the head. In severe cases, cyclizine hydrochloride (Marzine), 25–50 mg. t.d.s. may be given, except in pregnancy. The symptom usually subsides within a few months.

IX, X and XI. The Glossopharyngeal, Vagus and Spinal Accessory Nerves may rarely be damaged by a fracture involving the jugular foramen.

XII. Hypoglossal Nerve injury is extremely rare indeed.

Chapter 5

CONVALESCENCE, REHABILITATION AND SEQUELAE

Convalescence and Rehabilitation

Four Factors

The process of recovery in the uncomplicated, average case has been considered briefly in Chapter 3. The factors which determine whether or not there will be a smooth convalescence and return to work are numerous, and their inter-relationships complicated. They may be considered under four headings: *the injury*; *the patient himself*; *his occupation*; and *his domestic environment.*

1. The Injury.—It should first be mentioned that the degree of post-traumatic psychological disability is not necessarily in proportion to the severity of the brain injury. Often it is quite otherwise, in that a most severe neurosis follows an injury that was quite trivial (see p. 78). Nevertheless, it is important that an accurate assessment be made of both the general severity of the injury and the special effects that it has produced, because only in this way can the management of the case be other than empirical. The quality and quantity of both the physical results and the organic mental disturbances of the injury must be recognized, and it is here that neurology is of practical help to the patient.

Accurate Assessment

P.T.A.

As has already been mentioned, the P.T.A. gives some indication how long the patient will be away from work. When this is less than an hour, an early return can usually be expected.

One aim is to prevent the aggravation of untoward neurotic symptoms which may result from injudicious management: for example, by the bullying back to early activity of those who have suffered considerable, but unrecognized, traumatic subarachnoid haemorrhage; or, contrariwise, by permitting the recipient of a minor injury to be treated as a serious invalid for an inordinate period by well-meaning relatives, who may suppress a natural emergence of confidence and allow full play to any tendency towards neurosis.

2. The Patient Himself.—Here the complexities of *personality* enter with force; but *age* is also important. *Personality* It appears to be more difficult to get back to work a *Age* disabled man who has passed middle age than one who is younger. The power of *adaptation* to any resi- *Adaptability* dual symptoms and disabilities is clearly a most important factor, as is the intangible quality of *confi- Confidence dence*. There is also, of course, a wide variation in the reaction to the injury: a few are badly shaken by a *Reaction to* relatively mild physical trauma, while at the other end *Injury* of the scale, a certain type of man will remain stolidly unmoved by a more severe accident and will return doggedly to the saddle of his offending motor-cycle as soon as he leaves hospital. Most of us react in an intermediate fashion, which is, broadly speaking, consistent with the integrity and degree of vulnerability of our psychic constitutions, and here psychiatry succeeds neurology in helping us to understand and so to act appropriately.

3. The Occupation.—We now enter the field of industrial medicine. Generally, it is easier to get skilled or semi-skilled men back to work than the unskilled. Presumably, the same qualities that make a *Skill* man a skilled worker or not operate to make this so. This does not apply, of course, to cases where a physical disability itself is such as to prevent resumption of the skilled work.

Residual Disability

The exact nature of the work done should be discovered and related to any residual symptoms or disablement. Is the work manual or clerical? Is it noisy? (Many patients are unusually intolerant of noise for a long time after a head injury, and this is not due to hyperacusis.) Is working at heights involved for a man who suffers from vertigo? Does the work require special qualities of vision or hearing which may have been affected?

Attitude to Work

What was the patient's attitude to his work before he was injured? This is more difficult to discover, but it seems also to be an important factor in determining whether or not he returns to work readily.

4. Domestic Environment.—Over-solicitous relatives have been mentioned. The part of the spouse during the convalescent period is a highly important one.

The Spouse

A wife's (or husband's) own reaction to the injury and to any resulting financial stringency, and her confidence and adaptability, are all reflected upon the patient, who may be an irritable and awkward, and even a nearly impossible person to have about the house. The marriage vows take on a new significance, and the gear wheels of mutual adjustment may creak ominously, for this is not the individual she married. Many wives have said how changed their husbands have been, some for quite a long time; some, alas, permanently. The change may be in respect of quite small matters, which are nevertheless important in a home. Sexual relations may become strained owing to either increased or decreased desire or performance on the part of the injured one. Very little of these important aspects of the case is likely to emerge unless the spouse is specifically and separately questioned, when it may be discovered that a man who appears at a routine clinical interview to be normal is at home trying his wife's patience to the utmost. Great disharmony may ensue unless there is limitless tolerance during this difficult phase.

Separate Interviews

The normal noise of children seems to be a particular source of irritation to the sufferer, and it may be wise for the parents to lodge their children with relatives or friends if this can be arranged. Needless to say, the physical state of the living accommodation should be considered in relation to any of the patient's disabilities.

The Desirability of an Integrated Service

Some idea of the scope of these aspects of head injury work will have been gained when it is seen that social medicine is now involved, in addition to surgical neurology, psychiatry and industrial medicine, which have already been mentioned. It is not however usually possible to offer the patient more than a fragmented service from these different disciplines.

There is thus a very strong case for special centres for head injuries, where these various services can be integrated with the object of getting patients back to work as quickly and with as little economic loss as possible, just as, during the last war, such centres existed for the purpose of avoiding wastage of manpower in the Armed Services.

Rehabilitation Itself

A *graduated* return to normal activity should be the aim, and this ought to occupy the shortest possible time that circumstances will allow; for failure to start work at the optimum time may make it more difficult to do so later. There is one particularly tiresome circumstance which may work against a man who is fit and able to work, and that is when he is prevented from doing so because medical examinations and reports are first required, usually on account of litigation. These may cause considerable delay, during which boredom, inactivity and perhaps preoccupation with the apparent importance of such symptoms as are repeatedly elicited during these examinations may germinate the seeds of neurosis. It may be extremely

Rehabilitation versus Compensation

Justice

difficult both to effect a speedy and efficient rehabilitation and to do justice to any claim that there may be for compensation; for the two tend naturally to work against each other, and justice is usually a slow business.

Some patients will try to rush too fast towards recovery and, unless restrained, will invite discouragement. With others, it will be difficult to know just when or how hard to start urging them forward. The most difficult are those whose attitude towards their occupation was unsatisfactory before they were injured, and, if the injury was at work, what was originally a mild dissatisfaction may easily become an established grievance or grudge, and thence an open hostility, accompanied by a desire for compensation at all costs. Here, the subtlety of the disability and its subjectiveness may defy attempts at accurate assessment: the sufferer will not work until he has been compensated, and by the time he has been, perhaps after years of litigation, he is sometimes in no state to do any useful work again. Inactivity after discharge from hospital seems to be particularly erosive; few people seem able to keep in any sort of training for work while at home. Financial deprivation and uncertainty about the amount of eventual compensation only aggravate the demoralization that ensues, and post-traumatic neurosis is seen in its worst form.

During the latter part of convalescence, normally active brains should be reactivated, and usually active limbs exercised according to the skills that have been required of them. In hospital it is useless and perhaps frustrating to coerce into basket-making or rug-making an unwilling manual labourer who has no aptitude for that sort of thing, and who normally spends his spare time in the public house or watching television. But some sort of creative work ought to be available if possible for those who might wish to occupy themselves in this way, and the patient's own hobbies should be taken into account. The personality of the occupational therapist is all-important, and a pretty face may succeed in persuading normally indolent men into the most surprising pastimes.

Industrial rehabilitation centres can do much for those who have suffered disability and who genuinely wish to learn a new skill commensurate with their particular handicap, and great trouble is taken to try to launch them into useful and remunerative work. For those whose complaints are mainly subjective and for whom compensation is still unsettled, the rehabilitation centre is not normally a success.

One still meets with the old doctrine which insists that a man is either completely fit or unfit to do his original job, and on both sides in industry there are those who will not make allowance for the fact that an injured man often needs to start his old work *gradually*, in order to become fit eventually to do it with full efficiency. *The best form of occupational therapy is one's own occupation*, provided it is not an uncongenial one.

SEQUELAE

Following a mild or even a moderate head injury to a person who is psychologically robust there are usually few sequelae. On questioning, mild symptoms of the type which are heavily emphasized by those who suffer from neurosis may be admitted, but these are normally well tolerated and soon clear up.

The 'Post-Concussional Syndrome' and Accident Neurosis

Accurate definition is difficult, but it is convenient to attempt to separate these two conditions. The former may be regarded as a natural and not unusual sequel of cerebral concussion and contusion, a self-limiting period of symptomatology of variable degree lasting usually not more than a few weeks. The term 'accident neurosis', however, is used to embrace those patients who, without necessarily having been concussed at all, may have similar symptoms, but these are prolonged, exaggerated or elaborated and persist without relief usually until a compensation claim has been settled. On the basis of his wide experience, Dr. Henry Miller of Newcastle upon Tyne has given a most searching account of accident neurosis in his 1961 Milroy lectures*, and these should be read by all who wish to see the great complexity of the condition.

Miller points out that, for this neurosis to occur, the accident must fulfil two conditions: the patient must believe it to have been someone else's fault, and there must be a prospect of compensation. There is an inverse relationship of neurosis to the severity of the injury; neurotic sequelae are most frequently seen in unskilled or semi-skilled workers; there is an unexpectedly inconstant correlation with neurotic predisposition and scanty objective evidence of emotional disturbance. Last, there is absolute failure to respond to therapy until the compensation issue has beensettled, after which nearly all sufferers recover without treatment.

It should be emphasized that there is, understandably, a substantial amount of disagreement with Miller's views, and readers are urged to temper their enjoyment of his style with some of the robust scepticism that he himself shows towards the beliefs of his opponents. More recently†, his position appears to have hardened further, and he has come to regard accident neurosis as essentially simulation and malingering and as an index of the degree of the insurance and welfare services available.

The actual complaints are indeed subjective and frequently somewhat intangible in comparison with those such as anosmia or definite vertigo, which we can recognize as being organic in origin. There may be head-

* *Brit. med. J.*, **1,** 919 and 992, 1961.
† *Lancet,* **1,** 580, 1972.

aches of various types; persistent head pain localized to the site of the injury; 'lightheadedness' and 'dizziness', on which the patient may be unable to elaborate and which are not associated with particular movements or positions of the head (*cf.* p. 70, Fig. 8); lack of confidence; impaired powers of concentration; a lessened enjoyment of pleasures; and marital disharmony as the result of irritability, general intolerance or loss of libido. Minor defects of vision may also occur which cannot be attributed to any recognizable loss of visual acuity, visual field defect, or inefficiency of the powers of conjugate ocular movement, accommodation or convergence.

The pathological basis for this state is clearly a matter for continuing dispute and need not be further discussed here, except to say that one reason for regarding the syndrome as being basically organic in origin is the remarkable consistency of its general pattern in individuals of apparently widely differing psychological make-up. The stoic endures his temporary suffering with fortitude; while at the other extreme the sufferer from traumatic neurosis complains continuously and makes little effort to adapt himself until his compensation has been decided. But both at first have the same sort of symptoms, and the oft-quoted remark of Hugh Cairns puts the matter simply: "It is one thing to have a headache; it is another thing to complain about it."

The end result is determined *not only by the quality of the brain which has been injured and how much it has been injured, but also by the type of personality that has been affected and the degree of neuroticism*

Mention has been made several times already of the frequency of traumatic subarachnoid haemorrhage which may pass unrecognised. This condition has received little attention in discussions of the 'post-concussional syndrome', but it may well be relevant to the persistence of headache, particularly during the earlier stages of convalescence, for patients with spontaneous subarachnoid haemorrhage due to leakage of blood from 'berry' aneurysms may suffer similarly. Evidence that there is or has recently been blood in the c.s.f. can be obtained by lumbar puncture (p. 40).

Symptoms with a Recognisable Origin

Into this category fall symptoms and signs such as anosmia, blindness, hemianopia, diplopia, facial anaesthesia, facial paralysis, deafness, definite vertigo (p. 70, Fig. 8), limb weakness and dysaesthesia and ataxy, all of which are the result of specific neurological damage and which can be recognized by routine examination of the nervous system. Disturbances of speech, and difficulty in calculating, which did not previously exist, will also be elicited by simple tests (p. 14). Referred occipital pain may persist in patients whose pre-existing cervical spondylosis has been aggravated by the injury.

Dysphasia

Sufferers from dysphasia are sometimes thought to be demented, so that it is important to realize that there is not necessarily a loss of any faculty other than that of speech. That this may be so is illustrated by reference to no less an intellect than that of Dr. Samuel Johnson, who suffered from this disability for a short time as the result of a small stroke in the year before his death. Three days after the attack, he wrote about it to Mrs. Thrale as follows:

> "I was alarmed, and prayed God, that however he might afflict my body, he would spare my understanding. This prayer, that I might try the integrity of my faculties, I made in Latin verse. The lines were not very good, but I knew them not to be very good: I made them easily, and concluded myself to be unimpaired in my faculties.
>
> "Soon after I perceived that I had suffered a paralytic stroke, and that my speech was taken from me."

Some of these disturbances may not be appreciated by a patient whose insight has been blunted. In such a patient, intellectual impairment, personality changes, and the abnormalities of social behaviour that are associated particularly with bilateral frontal lobe damage will be revealed by the spouse or relatives if information is sought.

Traumatic Epilepsy

The incidence of this serious sequel to a head injury is a complicated matter which has been the subject of an extensive statistical study by Jennett (1962),* whose findings may be summarized as follows:

(a) Late traumatic epilepsy (the occurrence of even a single fit more than one week after a head injury) has an incidence of about 5 per cent for all cases of blunt head injury if they are followed for more than four years, but the risk varies widely in different types of case.

(b) Between a quarter and a third of patients who have had early epilepsy (within a week of injury), and a similar proportion of those who have had an intracranial haematoma, develop epilepsy later.

(c) Depressed fracture increases the risk in adults only if there has been early epilepsy or if the P.T.A. has exceeded twenty-four hours. The risk in such cases is about 50 per cent, but dural penetration further increases this risk in such predisposed patients.

(d) The risk of late traumatic epilepsy is only about 1 per cent for all injuries uncomplicated by early epilepsy, intracranial haematoma or depressed fracture, even when the P.T.A. is of more than twenty-four hours' duration.

(e) Although just over half of the patients with late

* Jennett, W. B. (1962). *Epilepsy after Blunt Head Injuries.* London: Wm. Heinemann Medical Books.

epilepsy have their first fit within a year of injury, this is delayed beyond the fourth year in more than a quarter of cases. (This is clearly of considerable importance in compensation cases which are usually irrevocably settled within this period of time.)

(f) Traumatic epilepsy is often severe and persistent, no matter what kind of injury it follows or after what interval it appears.

(g) The electroencephalogram is of no help in predicting the likelihood of this complication.

The impression that the clinician gets of the frequency of post-traumatic epilepsy is usually one of a figure that is too low, because the significance of isolated, sporadic or atypical attacks may be lost on the patient and his household, while some that are recognized may, for understandable reasons, not be revealed even to the medical practitioner. The concealment of epilepsy seems to be an increasing problem now that so many earn their living by driving or gain pleasure or convenience from motor vehicles. Occasionally, a patient will hide the fact that he had fits before the accident in order that the injury may be blamed for those occurring afterwards. Furthermore, when a fit occurs some years after an injury, particularly if it has been a mild one, a connexion between the two may not be appreciated either by patient or doctor.

Treatment.—Routine prophylaxis is unnecessary, but it is advisable to offer some protection against fits to those particularly at risk. Severely injured patients and those with depressed fractures, penetration of the brain, or intracranial haematomas should receive phenobarbitone, 30 mg. twice daily for at least six months after injury, reducing this to half the dosage for two weeks before discontinuing it altogether. There is a risk of precipitating fits by withdrawing this drug suddenly, particularly if it has been taken in larger doses.

For patients who have had even a single fit at any time after injury it is a matter of finding the medicinal régime which suits them best, for individuals vary greatly in their requirements. Anticonvulsant therapy should be 'tailor-made' rather than 'off-the-peg'. It may be necessary to try two or even three drugs in combination and permutation; phenobarbitone, phenytoin sodium (Epanutin), and primidone (Mysoline) are perhaps still the most useful. It is usual first to try phenobarbitone, 30 mg. thrice daily and then, if necessary, to add phenytoin, 50–100 mg. with each dose of the former. After this, primidone, 250 mg. three or four times may be tried alone, or in combination with phenytoin. There may be some initial intolerance to either phenobarbitone or primidone, but individually these are usually extremely safe drugs for prolonged administration. Phenytoin may, however, produce an unsightly hypertrophy of the gums in time, occasionally intoxication of the cerebellar system, and rarely a megaloblastic anaemia from interference with folic acid metabolism.

Late Meningitis

Patients who have sustained meningeal tears in relation to fractured air sinuses may suffer attacks of meningitis many years after the injury. This cause of pneumococcal meningitis, particularly if it is recurrent, should be remembered; for the extent of the original injury may have passed unrecognized, and its connexion with the subsequent meningitis is easily overlooked.

Inquiry may reveal that there have been bouts of rhinorrhoea, thought to be unusually "runny colds". Appropriate x-rays will usually indicate the fractured sinus and, after recovery from the meningitis, the patient should be referred for neurosurgical repair of the defect.

Retrospective Assessment

It may be useful to refer to the examination, usually for medico-legal purposes, of a patient who has sustained a head injury several months or even a year or two earlier. It will be realized that it is now somewhat easier to evaluate the case than it was soon after the injury; for at this late stage a panoramic view is obtained in which the changing picture can be more easily appreciated.

The chief requirement is a most careful history, which is usually time-consuming because of the desirability to have also the spouse's or relative's account and help in assessing symptomatology and supplementing the general account of a patient whose memory and perception may be defective.

Retrograde and post-traumatic amnesia should be carefully estimated, and it is surprising how easily this can be done in most cases, even when quite a long time has elapsed since the accident. Evidence of meningism in the early stages should be sought: was there neck stiffness, photophobia or persistent headache? Was convalescence smooth? How long did it take to get back to work, and if a long time, why? What was the patient's attitude towards his job before and after the accident? What residual symptoms are there? (direct, detailed questioning should follow the patient's spontaneous answer here). Have there been episodes of disturbed consciousness at all? A full neurological examination and a local examination of the injured area should follow, together with an evaluation of the general physical and mental health.

Summary

In conclusion, a restatement will be made of some of the more important principles mentioned in this chapter.

(1) Convalescence and rehabilitation should be con-

sidered in relation to the injury, the patient himself, his occupation and his domestic environment.

(2) Age, skill and attitude to work are important factors in determining how readily a man returns to work after a head injury.

(3) The degree of neurosis in candidates for compensation is often inversely proportional to the severity of the brain injury.

(4) The type of personality reacting to the brain injury is just as important as the quality of the brain and how much it has been injured.

(5) "It is one thing to have a headache; it is another thing to complain about it."

(6) The best form of occupational therapy is usually one's own occupation, provided it is not an uncongenial one.

APPENDIX 1

LOST BOUQUETS

by Brian Elliott

I lost my sense of smell as the result of a head injury. That was two years ago and I'm still without it, still searching for a word to describe the absence of the God-given faculty without which the rose and the hyacinth are robbed of half their beauty. For the first time I realised that we have no word in English to express the loss of smell, as "blind" and "deaf" express the absence of sight and hearing. Perhaps this lacuna in our language reflects the general opinion of people that the loss of smell is not grave enough to merit a name to itself.

My loss is not a major catastrophe, but it is a loss that I feel. I have not yet got accustomed to living in my odourless, scentless, smell-less world. It has its advantages, I admit. I could spend a day forking silage or cleaning sewage without noticing the stench. But I don't normally engage in that sort of work and my contacts with nauseating smells in the past were limited to an occasional gust from a stuffed drain or an open dump. While reckoning my immunity to unpleasant smells on the credit side, I find that it is more than outbalanced by my divorce from a wide range of smell-sensations connected with some of the most enjoyable things in life.

I mentioned roses and hyacinths. I could never resist the impulse to smell a beautiful rose. I would cradle the rich-scented blossom in my hand while inhaling the ethereal essence of its silky petals. A walk in the hospital garden one sunny morning cured me of the habit. Unthinking, I stooped to capture the fragrance of a particularly lovely rose. In one unforgettable moment came the stab of realisation that for me the scent of roses could never again be more than a memory. A part of me was dead. Shakespeare's words were painfully applicable:

> "*You smell this business with a sense as cold*
> *As is a dead man's nose.*"

Formerly I had been very sensitive to the smell of things. Memories of days gone by and of places far away were enshrined in their own particular aroma. The whiff of peat smoke rising in the cool air of evening evoked in me something of the nostalgia felt by Odysseus for his native Ithaca, and in my mind's eye I saw the blue wreaths drifting up from the friendly homes of Ballyshannon on the Erne.

The smell of beeswax always recalled the atmosphere of a certain Loreto convent where the parquetry owed its super-sheen to a home-made concoction of the butts of Mass candles mixed with turpentine. As a little boy with iron tips on my boots, I dreaded the perils of that polished floor more than the corrections of my veiled violin teacher.

Since those early days my museum of olfactory memories has been enriched with delights of many kinds. Eucalyptus oil has definite associations with chest-rubbing—a not unpleasant memory in itself. But to me it conjures up rather the picture of a sub-tropical garden near Baveno in Italy, where I plucked a leaf of eucalyptus and crushed it between my fingers. That was in 1947 and since then the fragrance of eucalyptus was linked in my memory with the smiling blue of Lake Maggiore and the terraced magic of Isola Bella.

If I could only smell a ship's hawser I would be wafted in memory once again to the scene from the rail of the "Tarkwa" tied up in Lagos harbour. The air is filled with a tangled web of odours. Cargoes of palm oil and ground nuts blend their earthiness with the tang of timber cut in equatorial forest and with the pungency of green oranges. The tray-loads of fish cakes balanced on the heads of the Yoruba women would have won a sniff in any ordinary Nigerian market; here even that doubtful savour is obliterated in the overpowering rankness. Certainly not a drawing-room atmosphere. There is a measure of relief in going to the other side of the ship and breathing in the brackish air of the lagoon.

My nose has always been partial to the bouquet of the vine, from the first crushing of the grape in a sun-drenched valley near Neuchatel, to the quiet dalliance with a glass of *vin rosé* in a lakeside inn at Zurich. I found the yeoman spirit of England preserved in the homely substantial smell of cider in the vat; I found the tang of Irish wit in the yeasty fullness of a pint of "Liffey water". But give me a glass of Hennessy and I am transported in thought to a mid-night scene at the airport of Castel Benito. Having flown across the desert I had exchanged some tattered Tripolitanian lire for a much needed refresher. The tawny liquid was welcome to my drooping spirit. Then I saw them, four of them almost ridiculously out of place, and yet nothing could be out of place at that airport where so many worlds meet. It was with unspeakable emotion that I gazed on those four Paul Henry pictures which brought a breath of Ireland to the sandy wastes of Africa. I shall never forget that glass of brandy. In it were blended the spirit of Champagne and the mystery of the Sahara and the opalescent blue of Connemara.

Arriving back in Ireland, my first meal was an Irish stew. I have my own hereditary formula for the perfect stew, but it does not taste the same just now. Returning home from work my nose was always alert to detect "what's cookin' ". I liked the smell of dinner to greet me at the door and had no time for those faddists who claim that the appetising odours of the kitchen should not pervade the rest of the house. If there's steak and onions on the menu, let it meet me at the garden gate! At least, that's the way it used to be. Now all those exciting tastes are scaled down and it is only after a few mouthfuls that they begin to register. Even a Chicken Maryland is somewhat insipid and a fried egg almost tasteless.

Recently I was doing some painting round the house and needed turpentine to thin the paint. There was a bottle in the basement cupboard, but I could not pick the right one from the array of unlabelled bottles of linseed oil, turps and varnishes. I cannot distinguish petrol from kerosene or lighter fuel, and I have to depend on the good little lady to prevent me having a first-class explosion with the blow-lamp. Janet, God bless her, has got accustomed to my "dead man's nose" and with her sixth sense she often comes to the rescue of my missing fifth. Poor girl, she knows I haven't the same interest in her cosmetic purchases. She misses my appreciation of her perfume, but then she's not the sort of wife who leads her husband by the nose!

I still have sight and hearing and touch and taste, and through these channels I can continue to draw upon the vast treasures of beauty in the world of nature and art and literature. But I miss the goodly smells of many things.

I miss the smell of the sea, and tang of the spray carried in from the wild Atlantic to Tullan Strand; I miss the warm smell of gorse in the hills above the Knather; I miss the smell of horses and dogs and all the mingled odours of life on the land. I smile upon the primrose and the violet; to me they are ever beautiful, but their beauty reaches me filtered of its lambent sweetness.

I still have the memory to cheer me. But memory itself is dimmed when the sense is gone, and only in my dreams do I sometimes recapture the vividness of the reality. A few nights ago I dreamed of lily of the valley and breathed its pure intoxication in my sleep. In the morning it was gone. I was back in my sterile deodorised world, whose roses—by whatever name—smell not at all.

APPENDIX 2

A System for Recording the Initial Examination of a Patient with a Head Injury

Name Age Occupation

History

Date Time of Injury
„ „ Admission
„ „ Initial Examination

Circumstances of Injury
Relevant Observations by Witnesses
Fits?
Alcohol?
Crash Helmet?
Seat Belt?

Examination

1. Adequate Airway? Shock or Haemorrhage?
2. Level of Responsiveness
   Alert, drowsy, or unresponsive (and to what stimulus)?
   Rational, orientated or confused?
   Length of Amnesia (if fully conscious and rational)
3. Neurological Examination, especially
   Pupils
   Hemiparesis, hemianopia or dysphasia? (R.- or L.-handed?)
4. Pulse, Blood Pressure, Respiration and Temperature
   (See also 1.)
5. Neck Stiffness and Kernig's Sign? Neck Injury?
6. Head wounds, bruising or oedema? (record carefully, with diagram). Blood or c.s.f. from nose or ears?
7. Other injuries?
8. Skull x-ray result

APPENDIX 3

A Specimen Observation Chart

Name   Age   Date of Admission

Date and Time	*Level of Responsiveness* (and other observations; e.g. fits, incontinence, vomiting, etc.)	*Pupils* (equality & reactions).	*Temperature*	*Respiration*	*B.P.* (systolic)	*Pulse*
28 June '60 9.00 a.m.	Responds only to painful stimuli by moving all four limbs naturally.	Right slightly larger than Left. Both sluggish.	98·0	28	150	70
9.30	Responds similarly. Restless. Vomited twice.	Equal. Sluggish.	98·6	24	140	90
10.00	Shouted, "Go away!" when shaken lightly. Restless.	Equal. Brisk.	99·0	22	130	90
10.30	Answers readily when name is called. Quieter.	Equal. Brisk.	99·4	20	130	85
11.00	Eyes open and taking notice. Answers promptly, but confused.	Equal. Brisk.	99·2	20	130	80
11.30	Less confused. Asked for urinal.	Equal. Brisk.	99·0	20	130	80
12.00 m.d.	More rational. Realizes he is in hospital.	Equal. Brisk.	99·2	20	130	80
12.30 p.m.	Knows what day it is. Remembers going to work on motor-cycle and then nothing more.	Equal. Brisk.	99·0	20	130	76
1.00	Rational, alert and correctly orientated.	Equal. Brisk.	98·8	20	130	74

(Uneventful progress and recovery).

Note the important place given here to the level of responsiveness and to the pupils. It is more than just a 'shock chart'.

INDEX